Heavily Tattooed
Men & Women

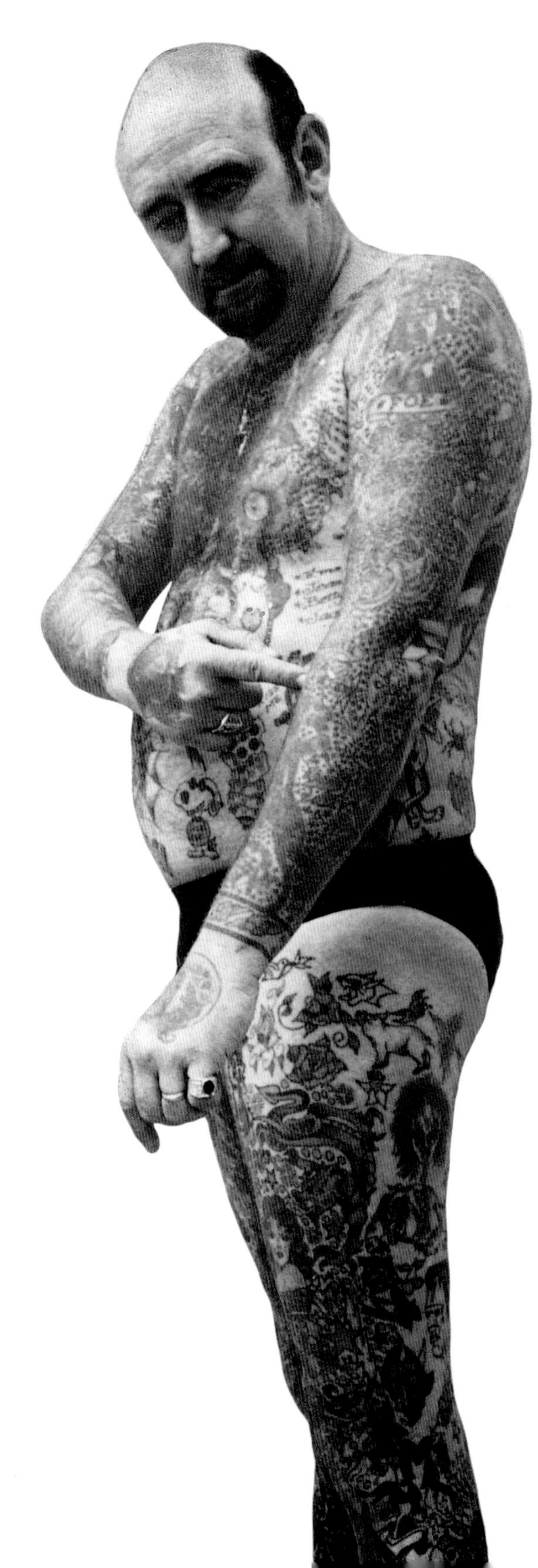

Heavily Tattooed
Men & Women

Compiled and Edited by
Spider Webb

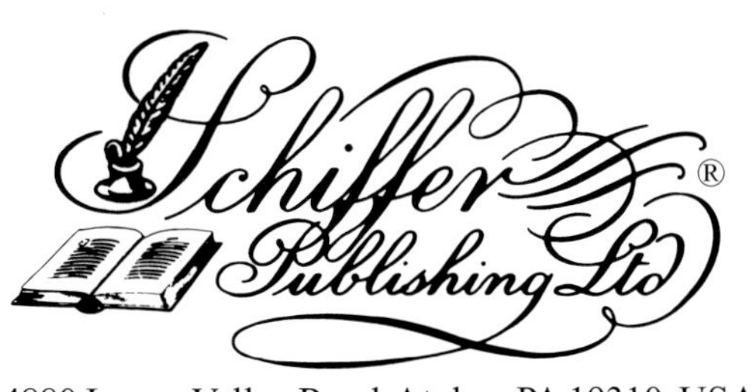

4880 Lower Valley Road, Atglen, PA 19310 USA

DEDICATION

For Tecla and the artists, models, and photographers of years ago who made this volume possible. Love and respect to you all.
Spider Webb, 2001

Cover photo:
Jean Carson, already highly tattooed, has more put on her leg by the greatly tattooed Charles Wagner as the famous Mildred Hull, tattooed girl, looks on. These three are very well-known among the tattooed people.

Back cover photo:
Photo of the author by SOS

Published by Schiffer Publishing Ltd.
4880 Lower Valley Road
Atglen, PA 19310
Phone: (610) 593-1777; Fax: (610) 593-2002
E-mail: Schifferbk@aol.com
Please visit our web site catalog at **www.schifferbooks.com**
We are always looking for people to write books on new and related subjects. If you have an idea for a book, please contact us at the above address.

This book may be purchased from the publisher.
Include $3.95 for shipping. Please try your bookstore first.
You may write for a free catalog.

In Europe, Schiffer books are distributed by
Bushwood Books
6 Marksbury Ave. Kew Gardens
Surrey TW9 4JF England
Phone: 44 (0)20 8392-8585; Fax: 44 (0)20 8392-9876
E-mail: Bushwd@aol.com
Free postage in the UK. Europe: air mail at cost.
Please try your bookstore first.

Designed by John P. Cheek
Cover design by Bruce M. Waters
Type set in Dutch801 Rm BT/Dutch801 Rm BT

ISBN: 0-7643-1605-2
Printed in China

PREFACE

attooing owes a massive debt to the invention of the camera, for by that means the most mortal of art forms can be preserved. The photographs in this book are part of my collection of heavily tattooed men and women dating from the invention of the camera to the late 1950s.

In many cases the photos initially served to illustrate a specific tattooist's work or as advertisements for those who chose to exhibit themselves in circuses and dime museums. Many were once sold individually to collectors of memorabilia on tattooing.

The collection these particular photographs are taken from was originally owned by Bernard Kobel of Clearwater, Florida, who amassed an enormous number of pictures over the years from numerous other sources, notably collectors in the unique and often hidden tattoo subculture (consisting of both the tattooed and people who, though not tattooed, are fascinated and often romantically or sexually attached to the tattooed human form). These collectors would exchange and donate photos among themselves the way others collect and trade stamps, coins, antiques, and art works. For years Kobel sold prints of his photographs by mail, and the title of this book, *Heavily Tattooed Men and Women*, was the title of Kobel's mail-order catalog. When he retired, I bought his collection intact to add to my already extensive collection of photos, designs, business cards, and other memorabilia relating to tattooing in all its aspects. After looking at the pictures, I was struck by the sheer waste involved in hiding them away in the dusty corner of a museum or limiting their circulation to a privileged few in the tattoo milieu.

As a tattooist and as an artist with a growing concern about the image tattooing has and the ignorance of the general public on the subject, I believe it essential to present the photographs in their correct context: as authentic examples of a living art—not an aberration of society.

Many of the subjects of these photographs chose total body coverage as a means of income—but by no means all of them did so. Their motivations are myriad and open to speculation as most are now dead. Standing alone, the photos speak for themselves; as a person who has many tattoos with numerous peers who do also, I hope that you, the viewer, can look at the photos with open eyes and be not too quick to judge the subjects as freaks first and human beings second. Human beings they are, and they differ from the norm only in that they made an incredible commitment. They chose a means of self-expression that entailed being labeled "freak" or "oddity" by those who tend to condemn what they cannot understand.

The names of the photographers, tattooists, and subjects have been kept anonymous. Most of their identities have been lost with time. The lives they lived and the art they lived with constantly speak in these photographs more clearly than any words possibly can.

Spider Webb
Mount Vernon, New York, March 1976

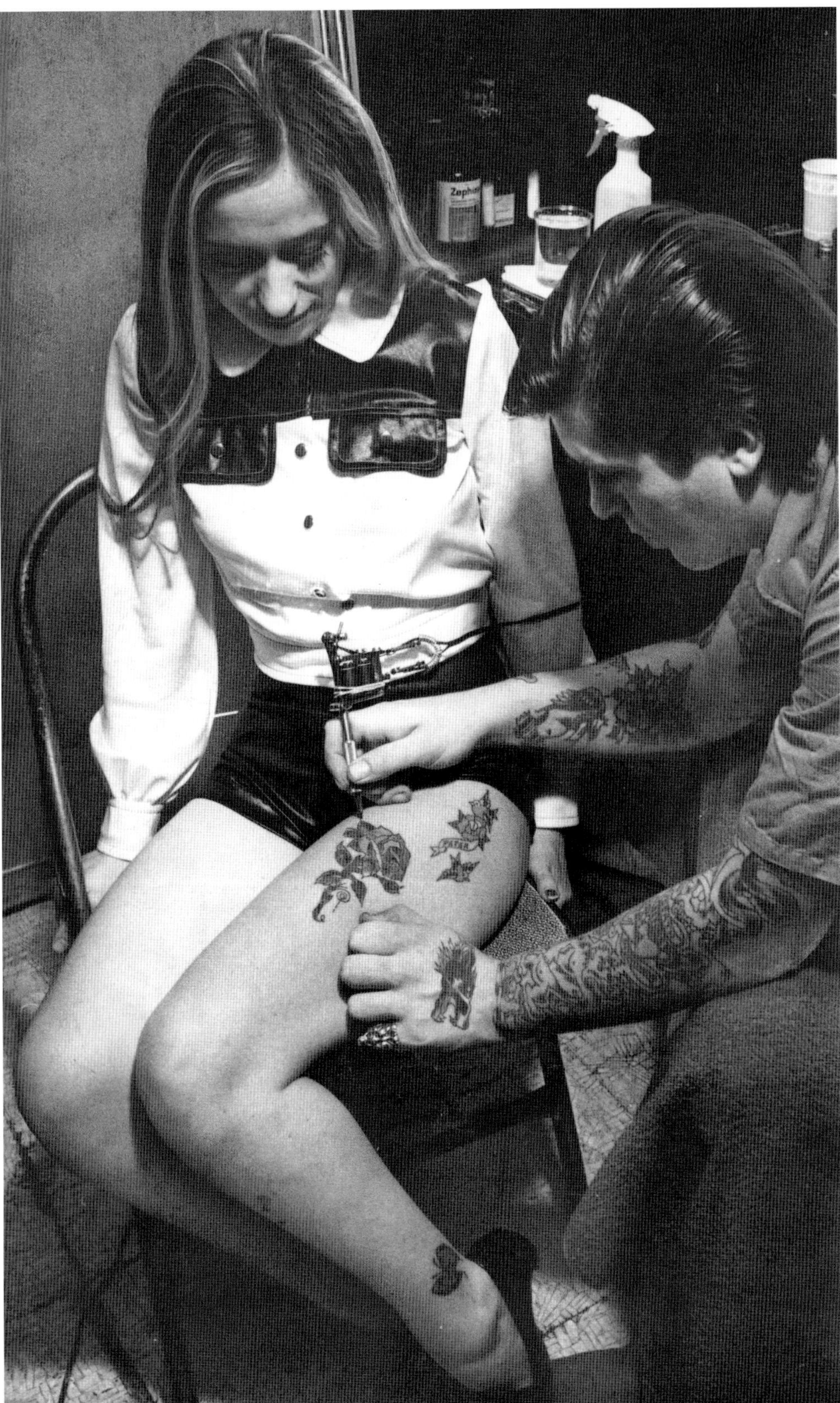

INTRODUCTION

1976. America's Bicentennial. It is hard to believe this book first came out twenty-five years ago this year. At the time, it was virtually the only book on tattoing available. If it is true that "every dog shall have its day," tattooing is now having its day: hundreds of books in print worldwide, thousands of magazines everywhere, museum and gallery shows, and people all over the globe wearing "warm" art.

I'm glad *Heavily Tattooed Men & Women* was part of this whole scene of change and it is nice to have it back again. Enjoy.

Spider Webb, New York City, 2001

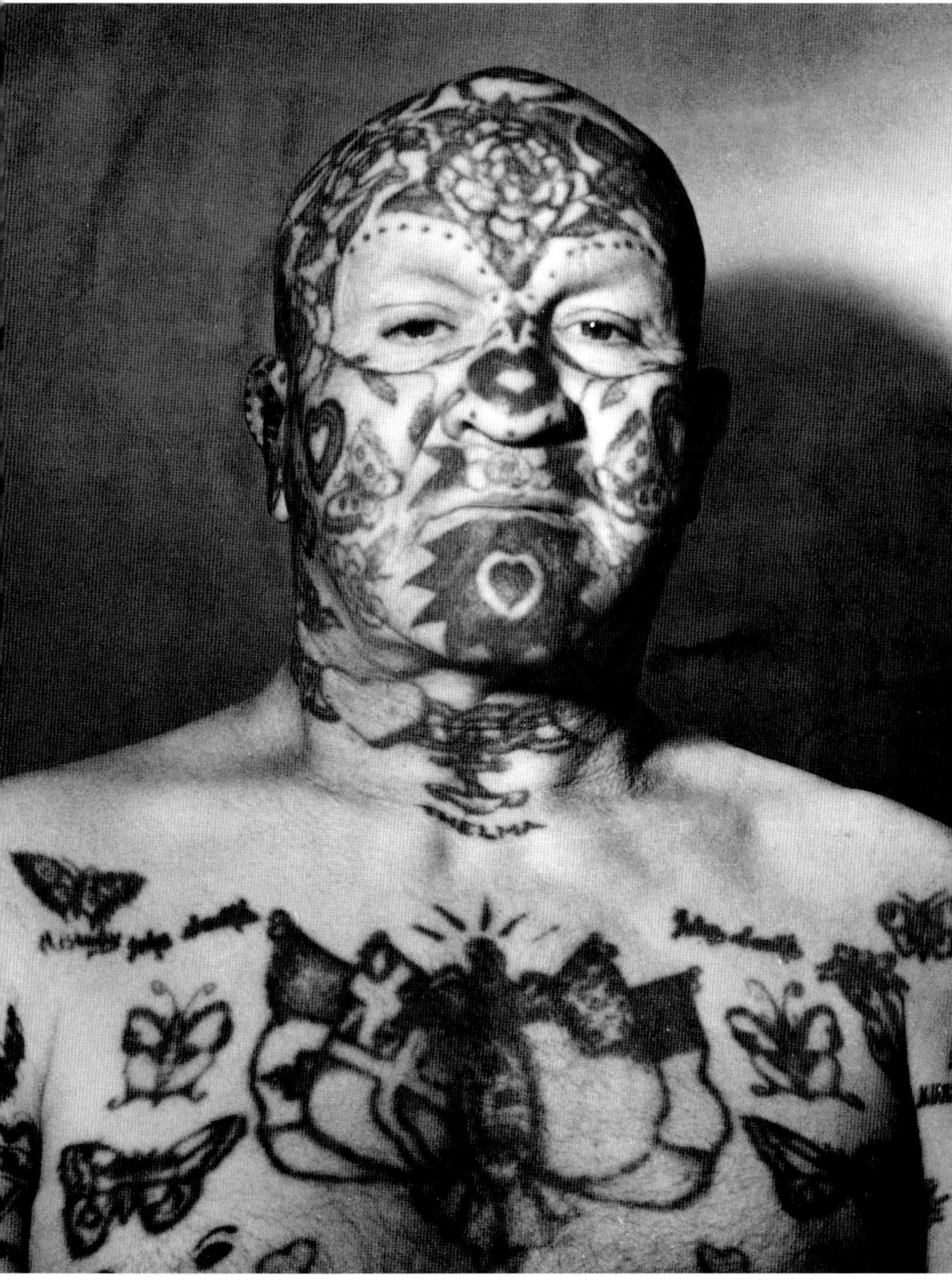

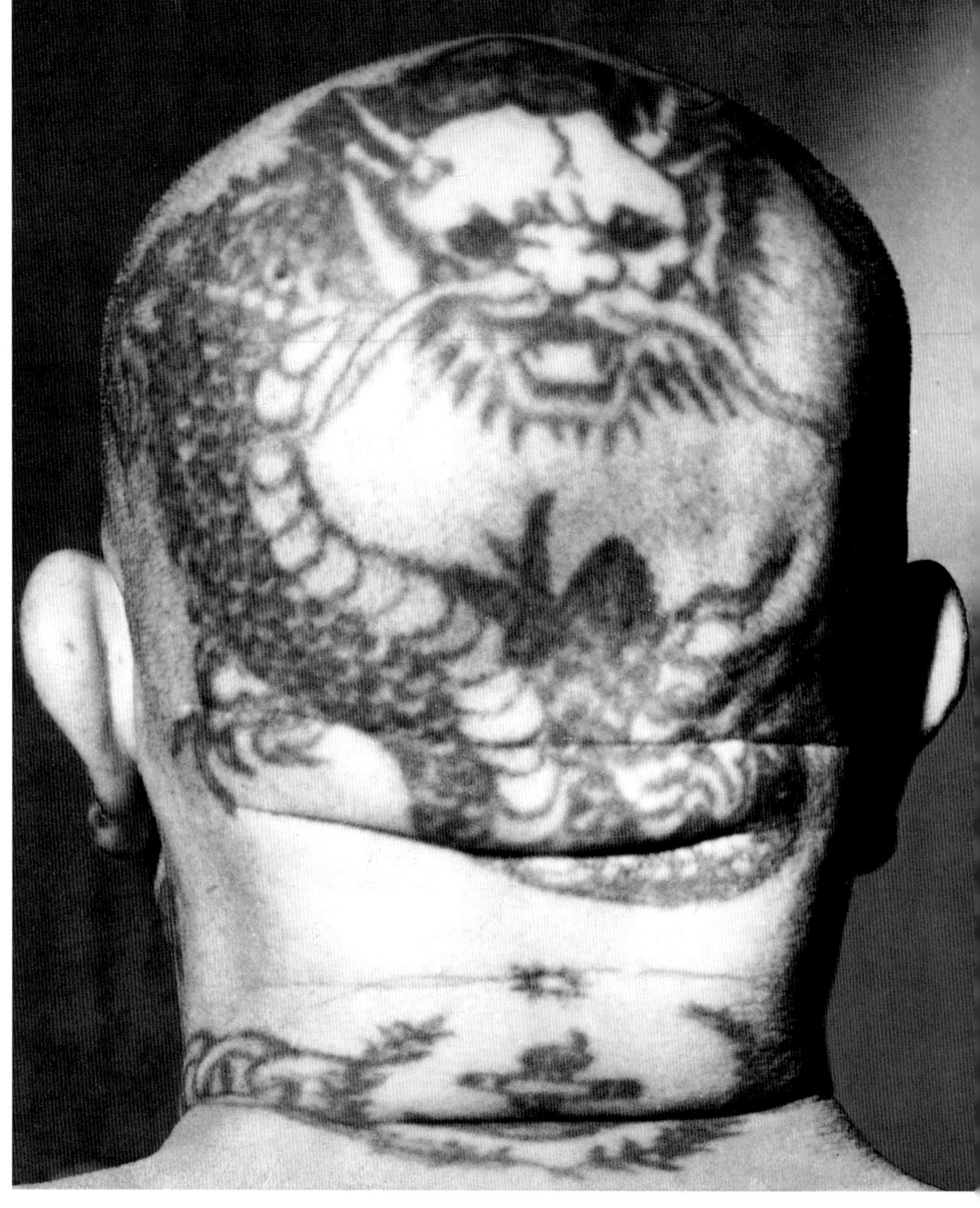

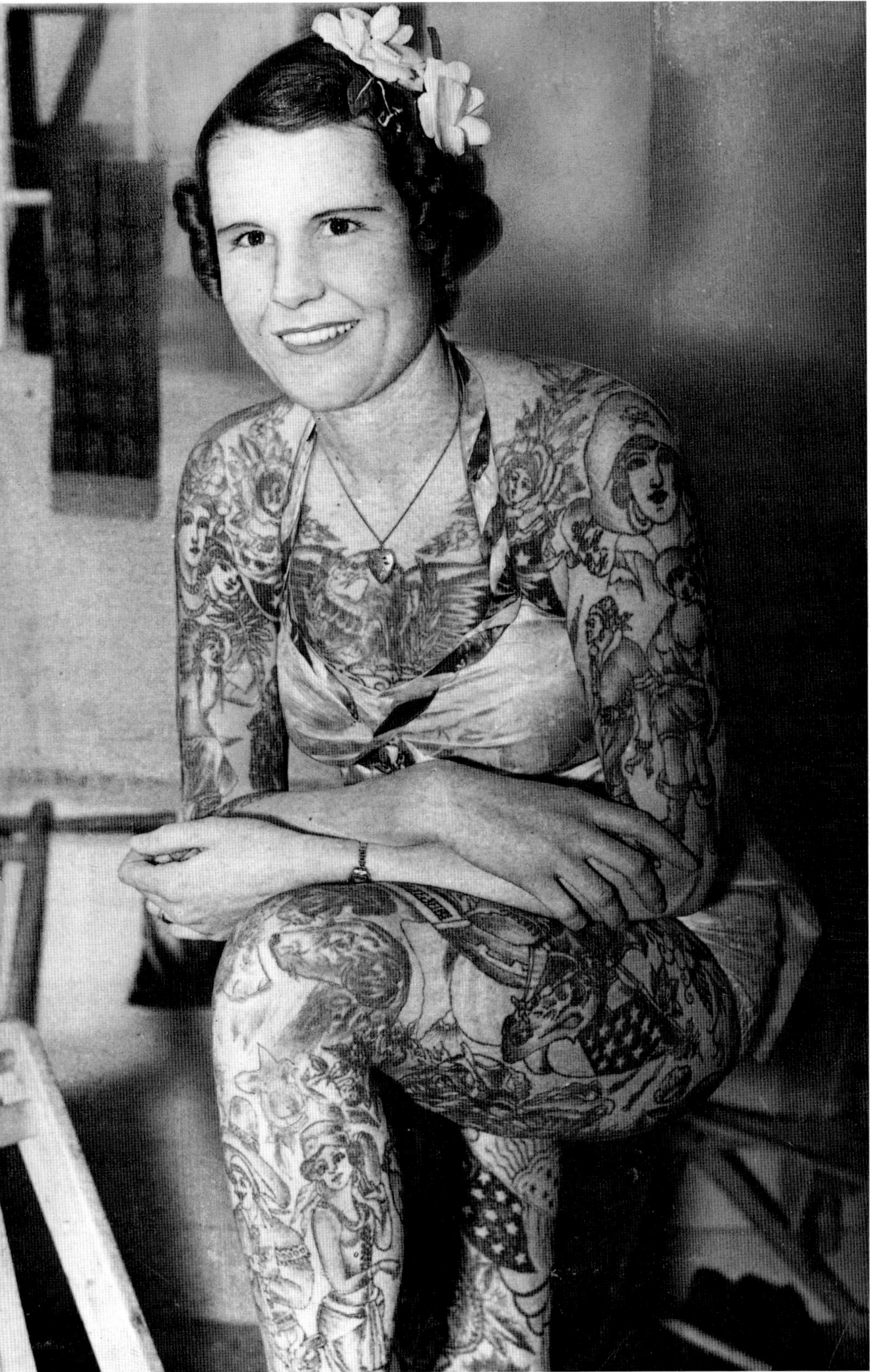

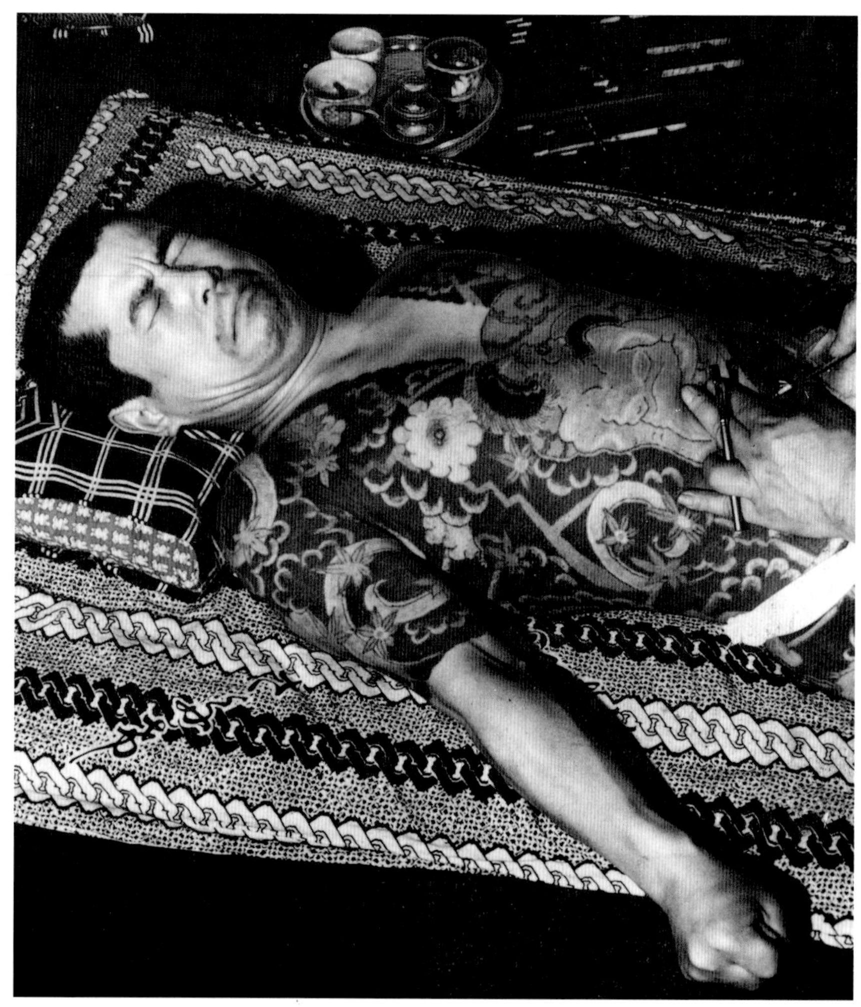

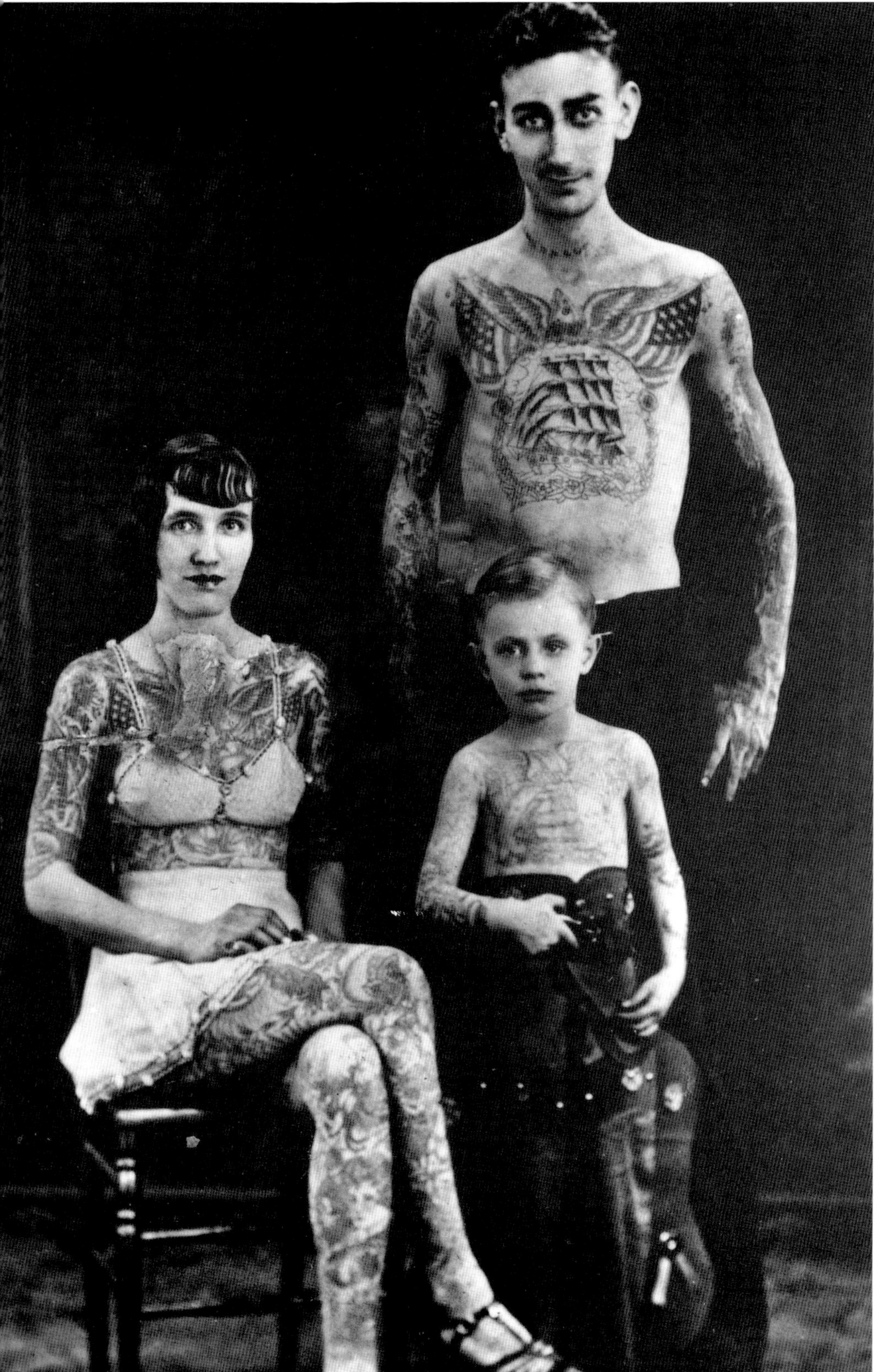

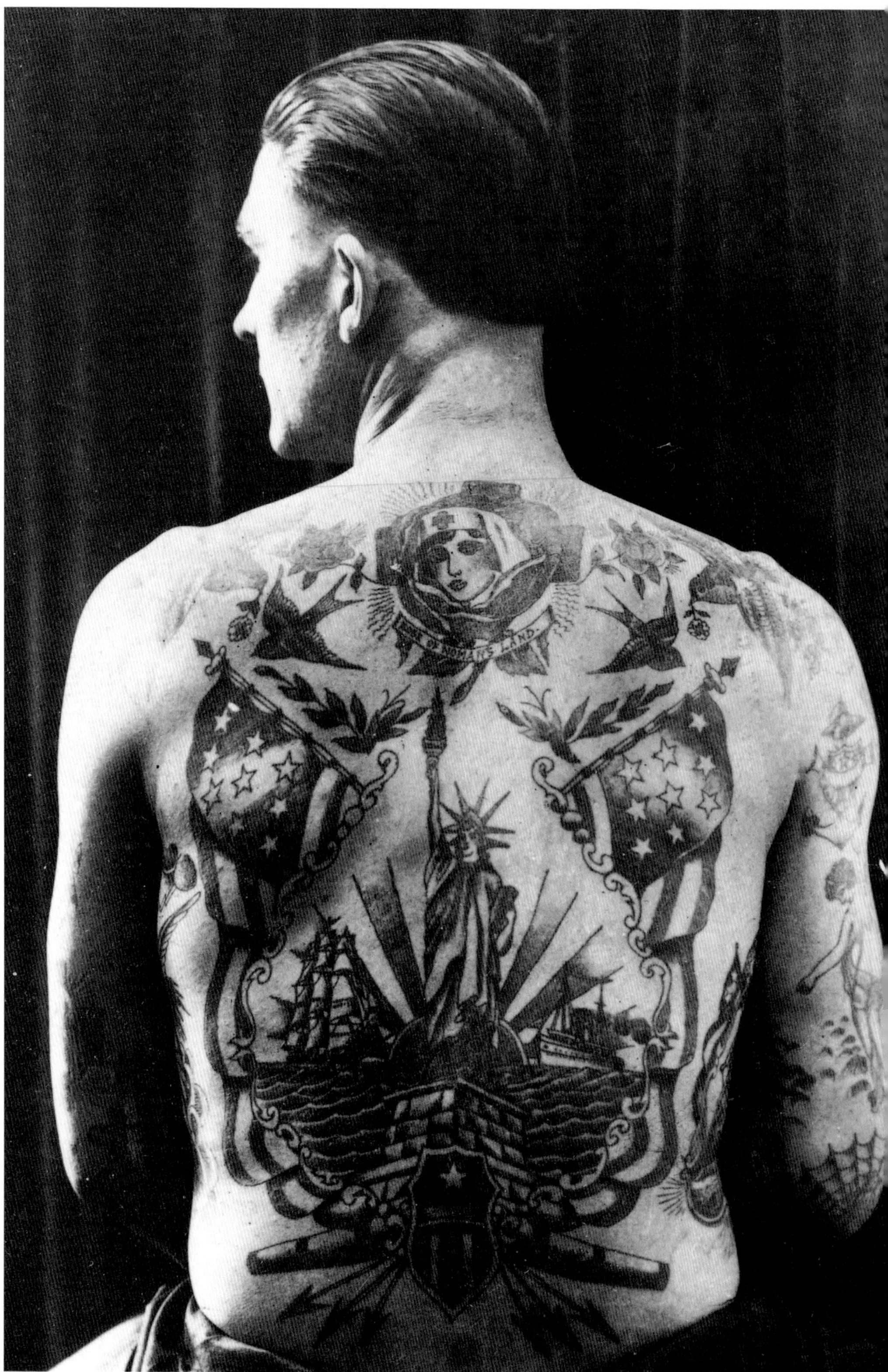
NO MAN'S LAND.

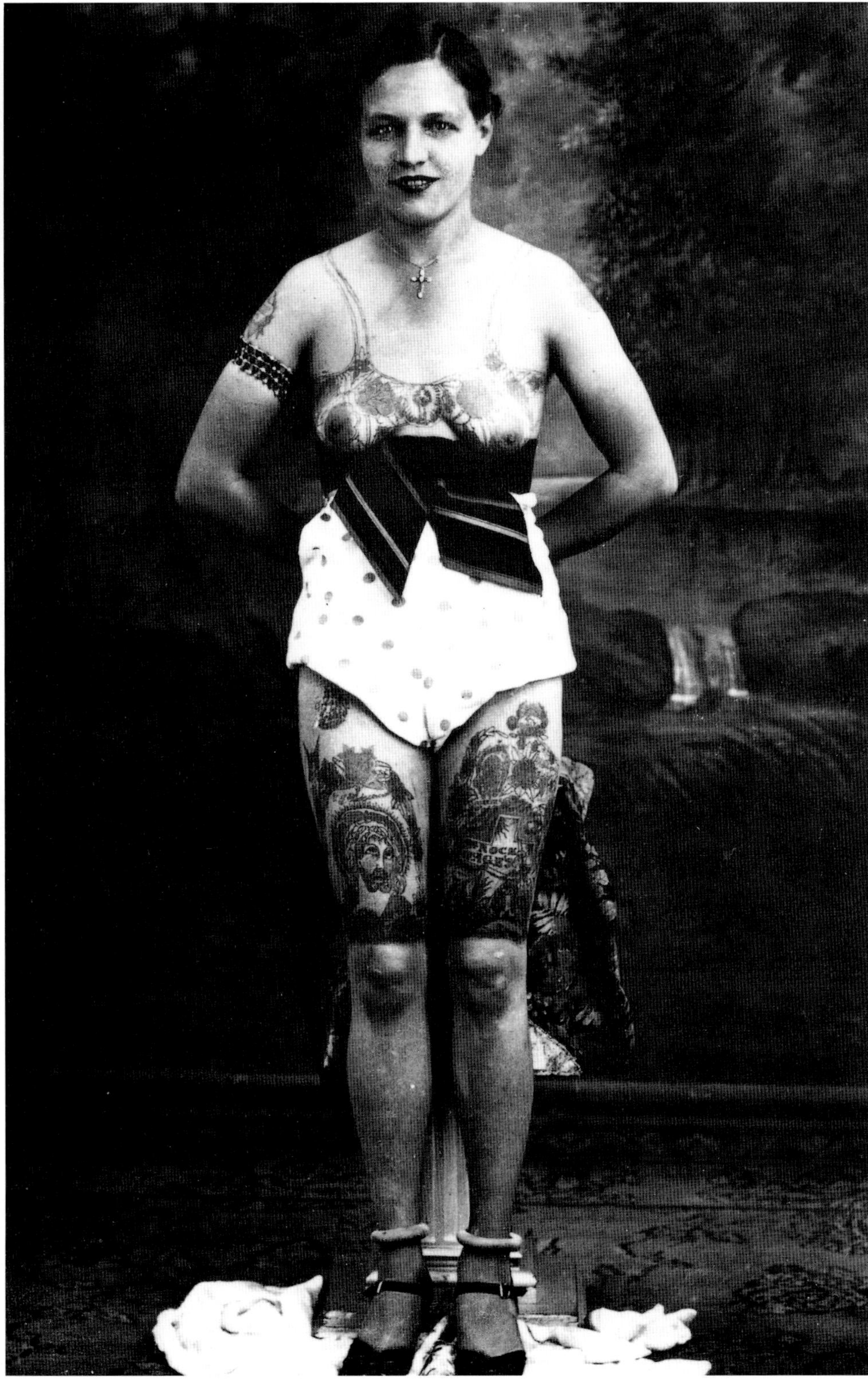

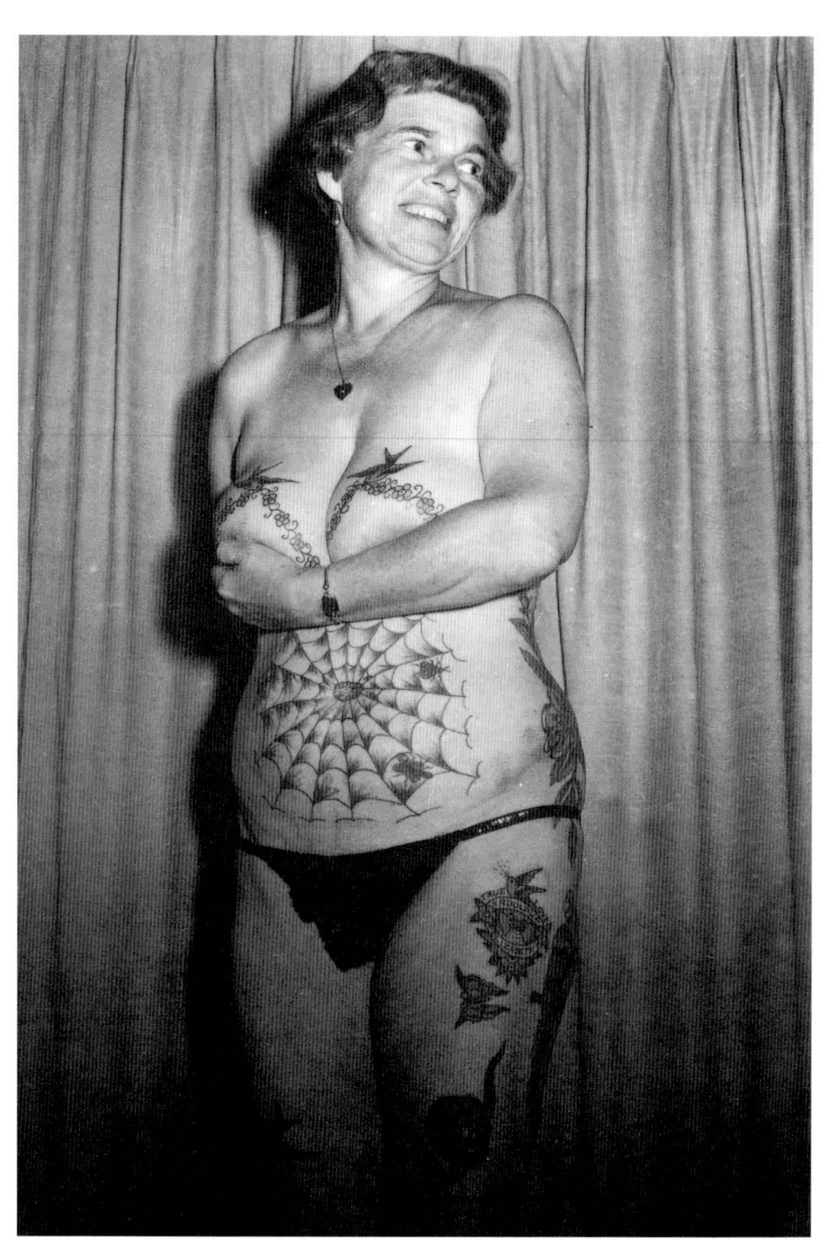

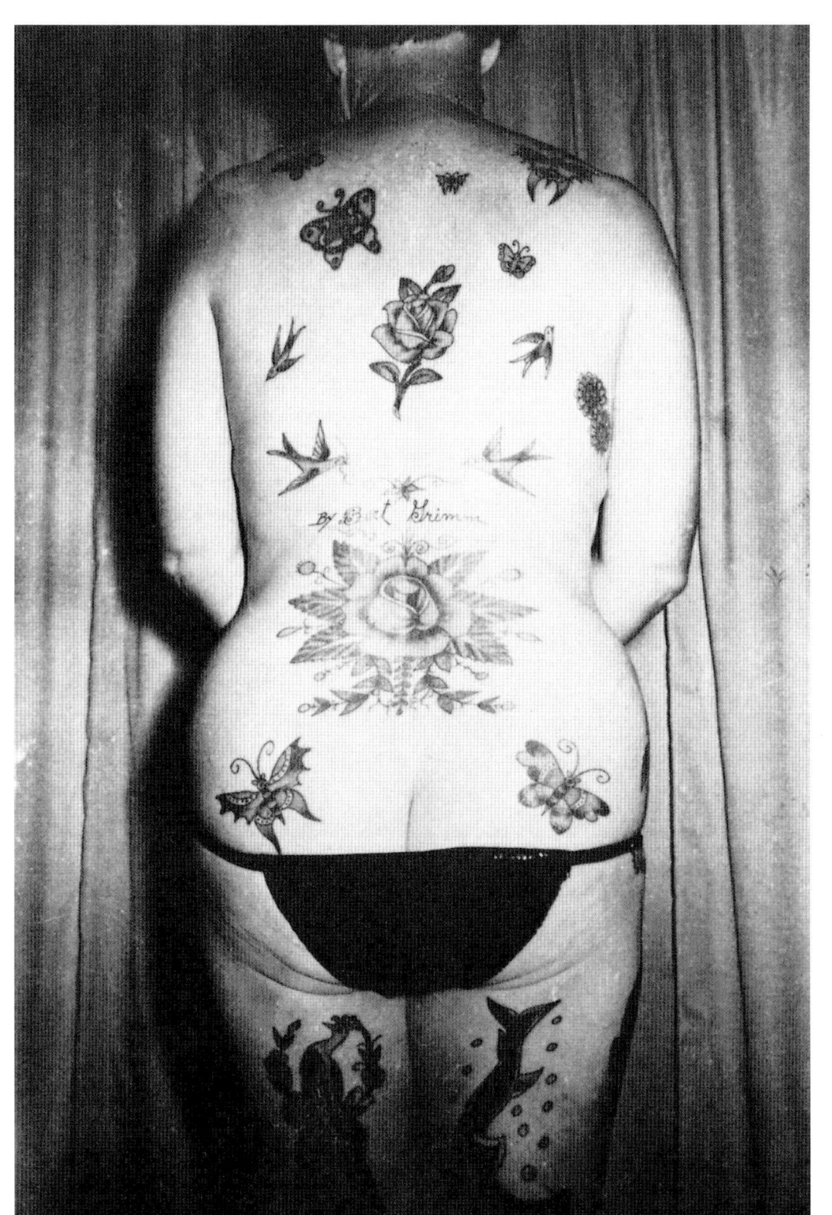

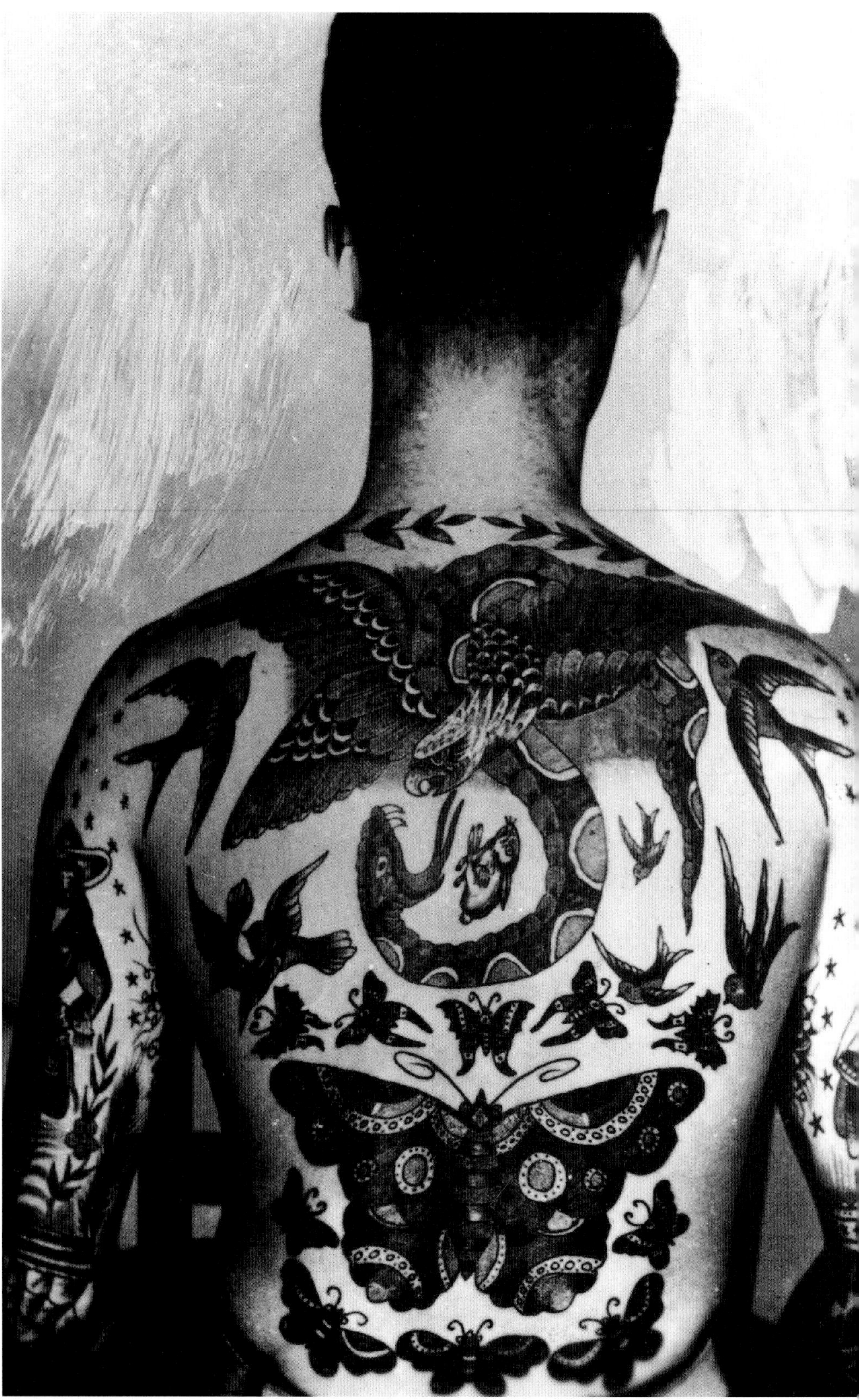

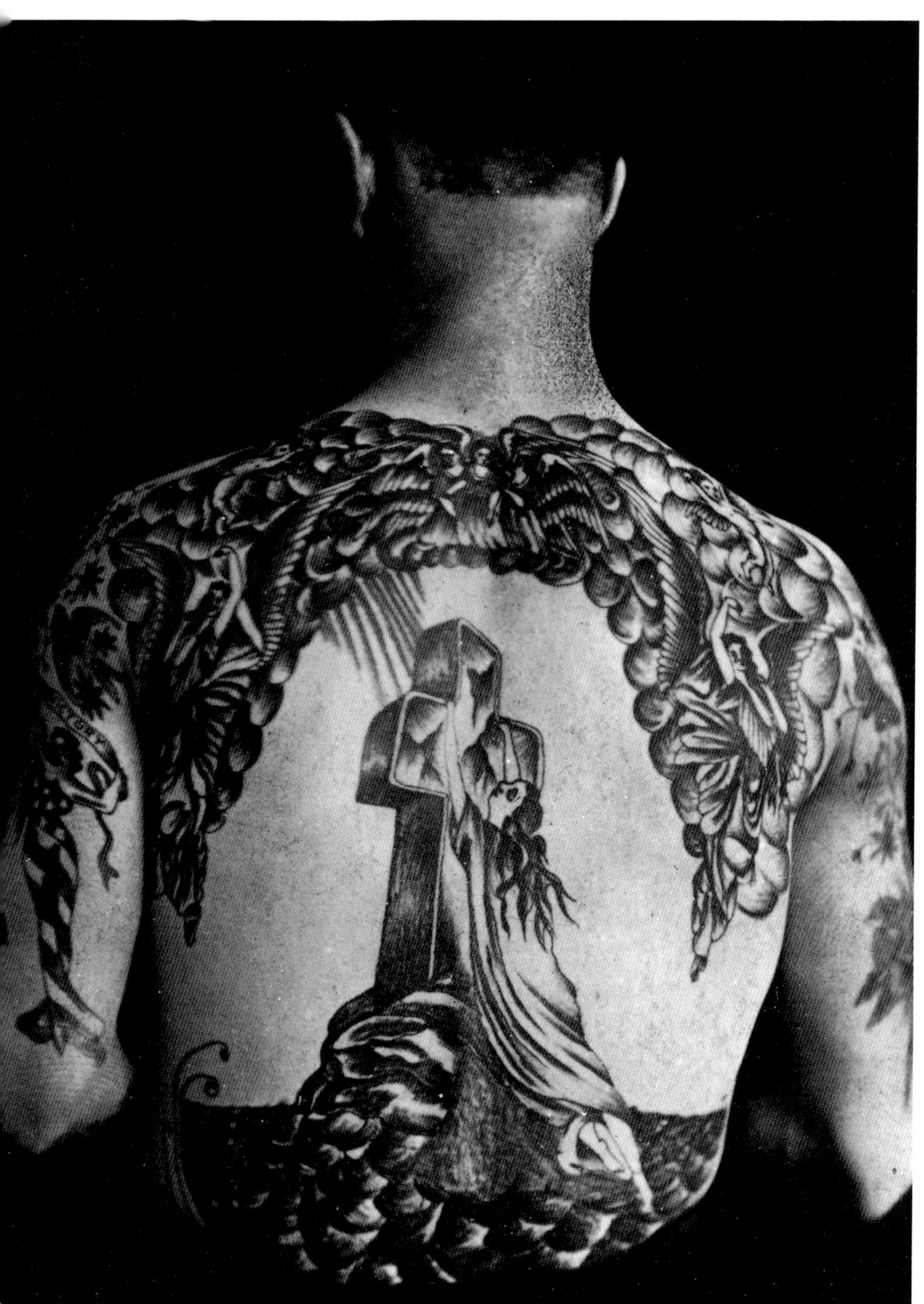

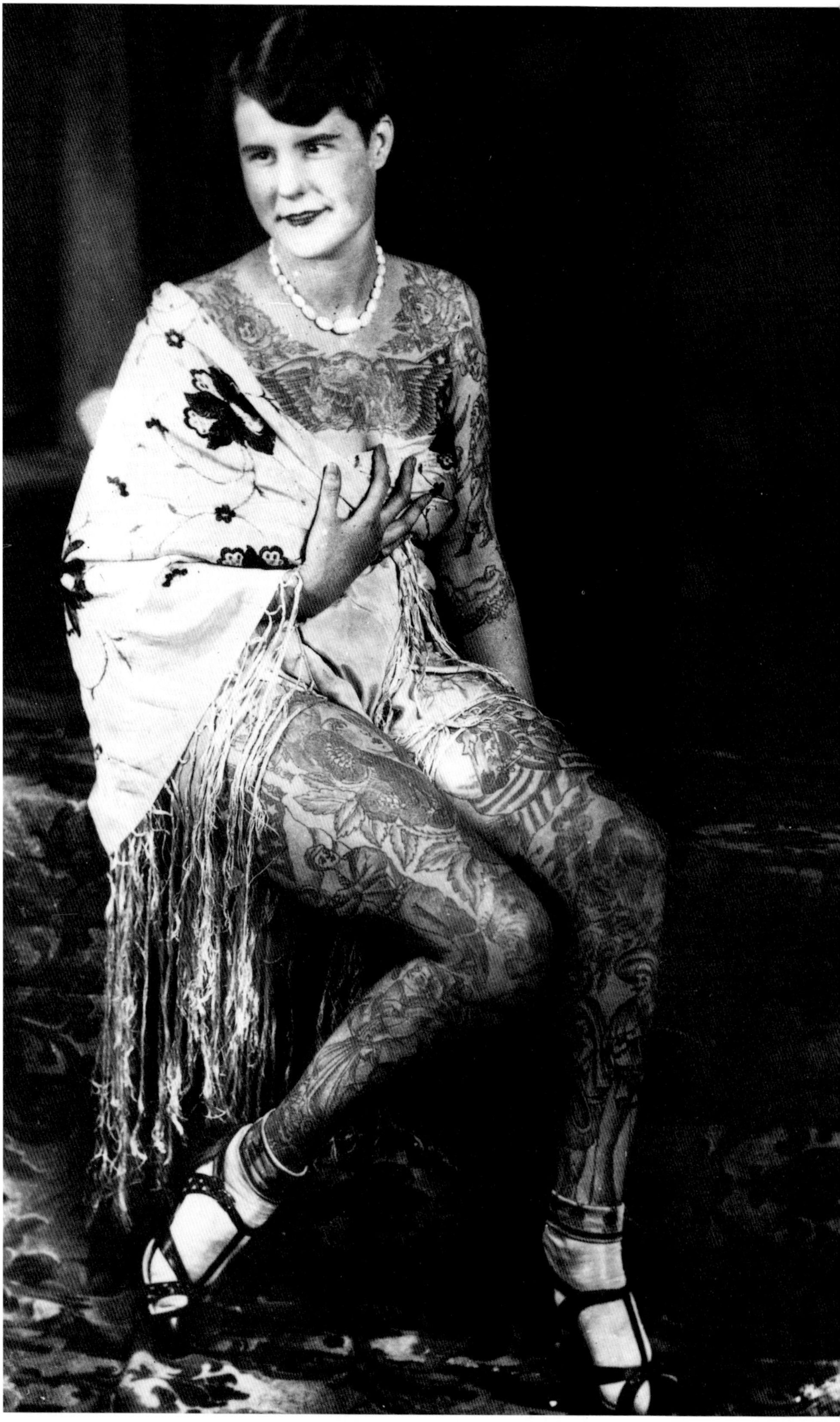

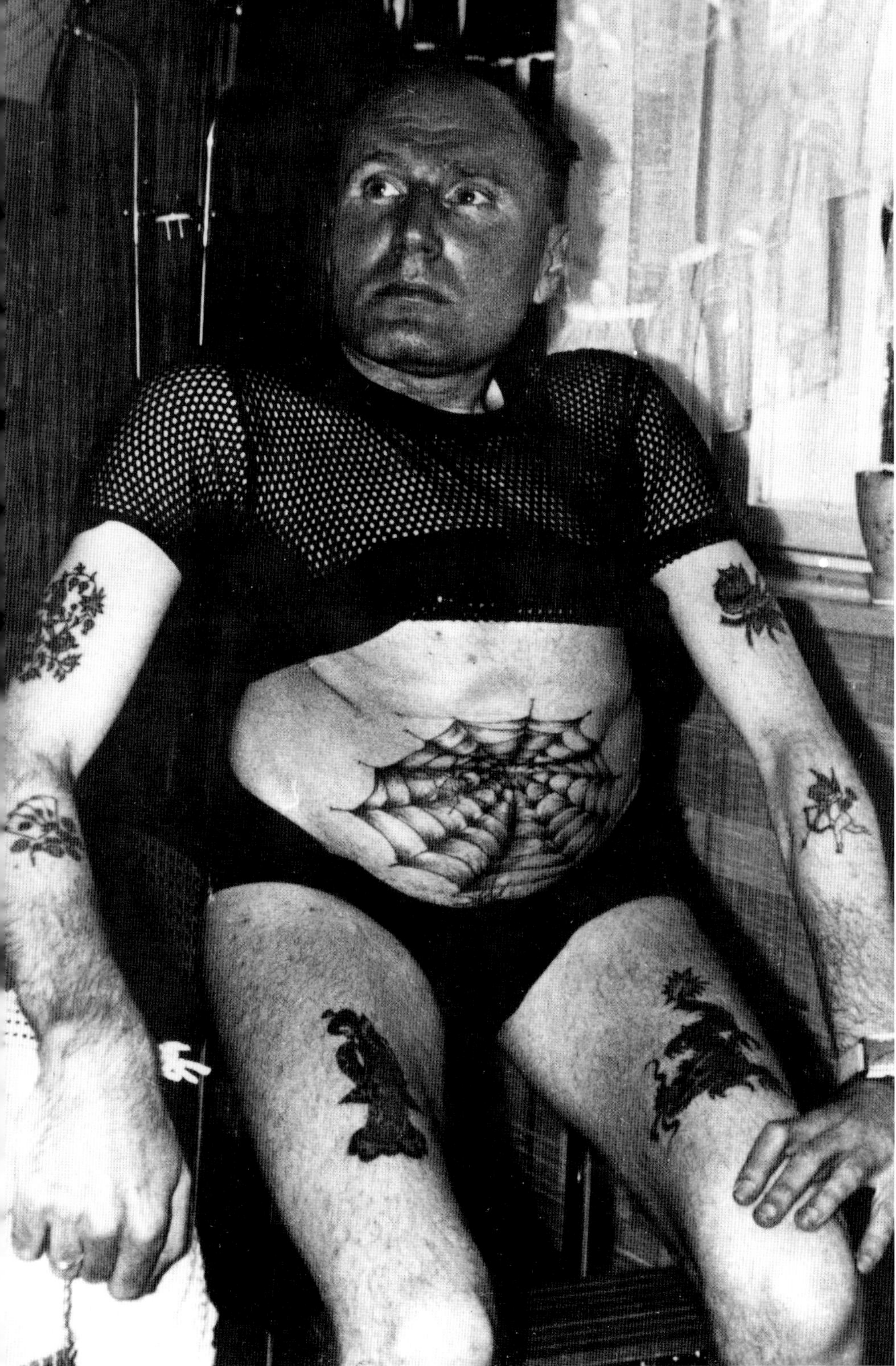

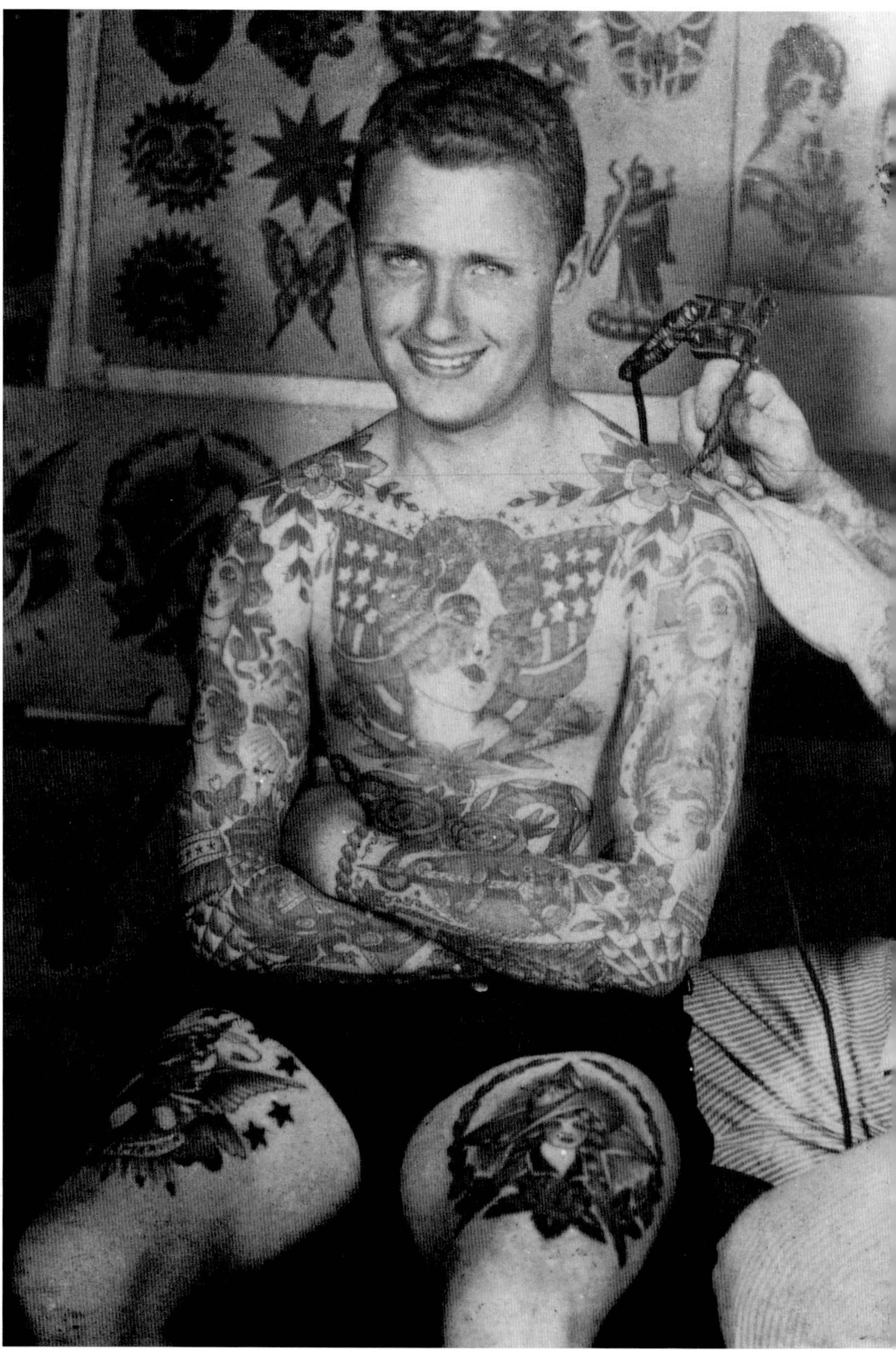

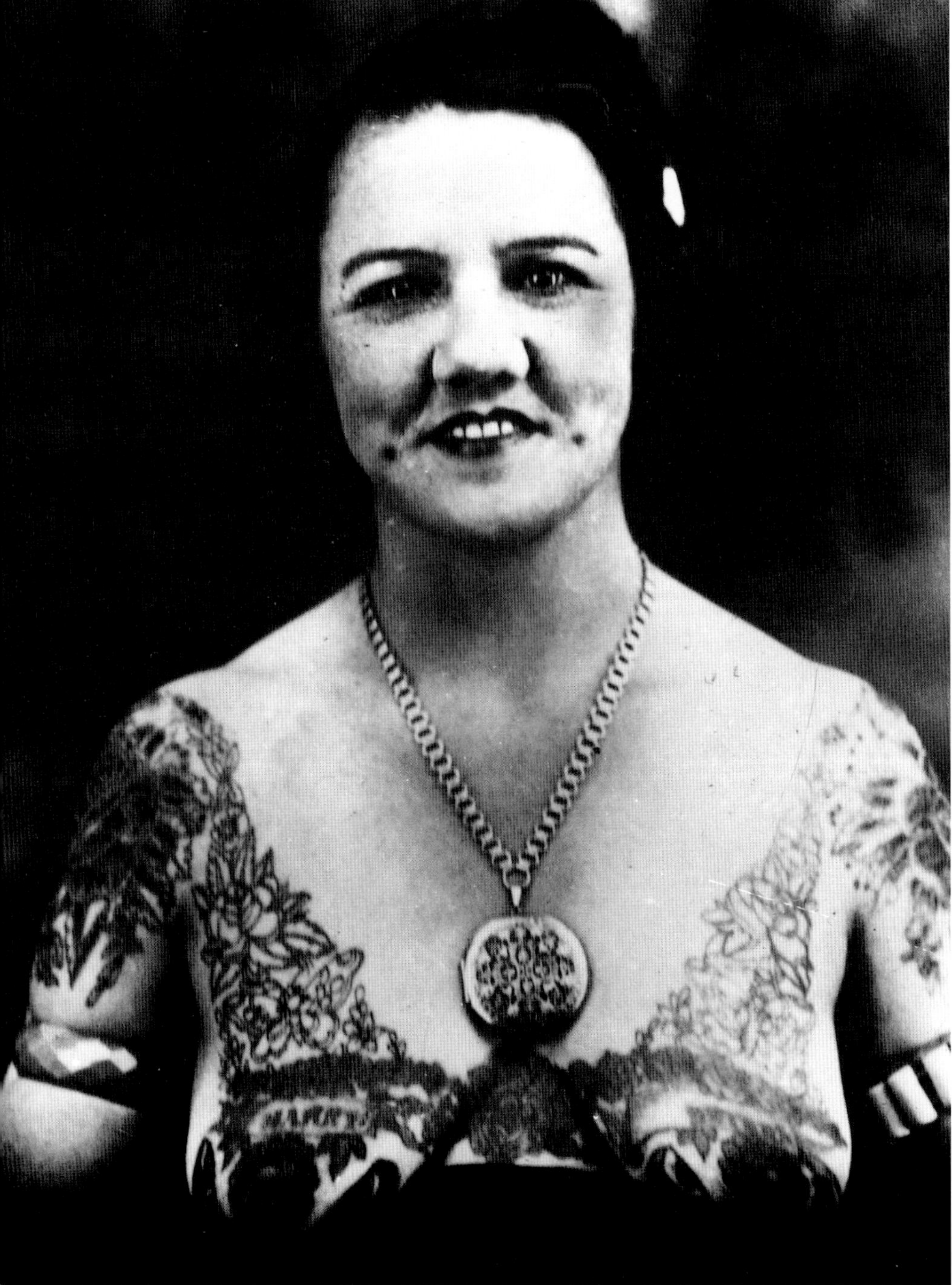

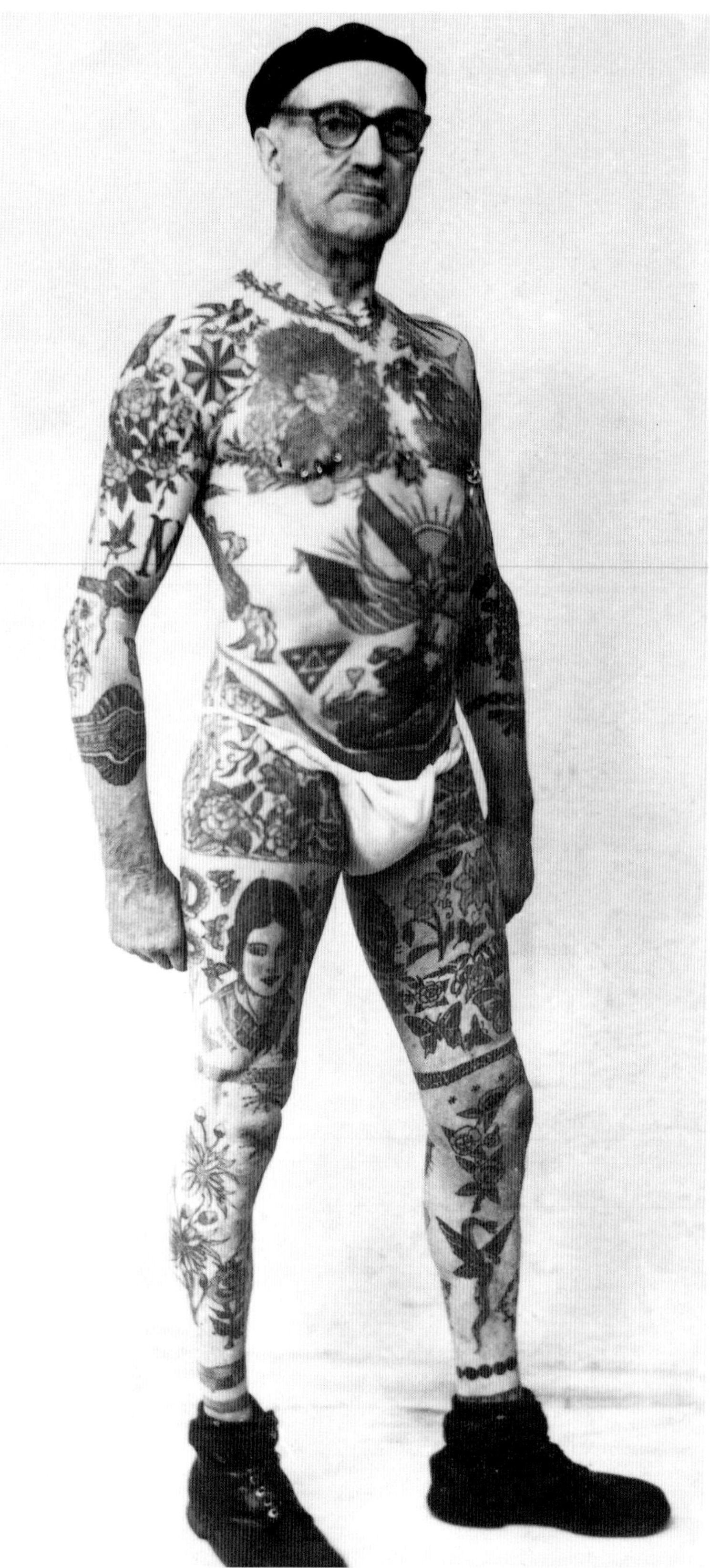

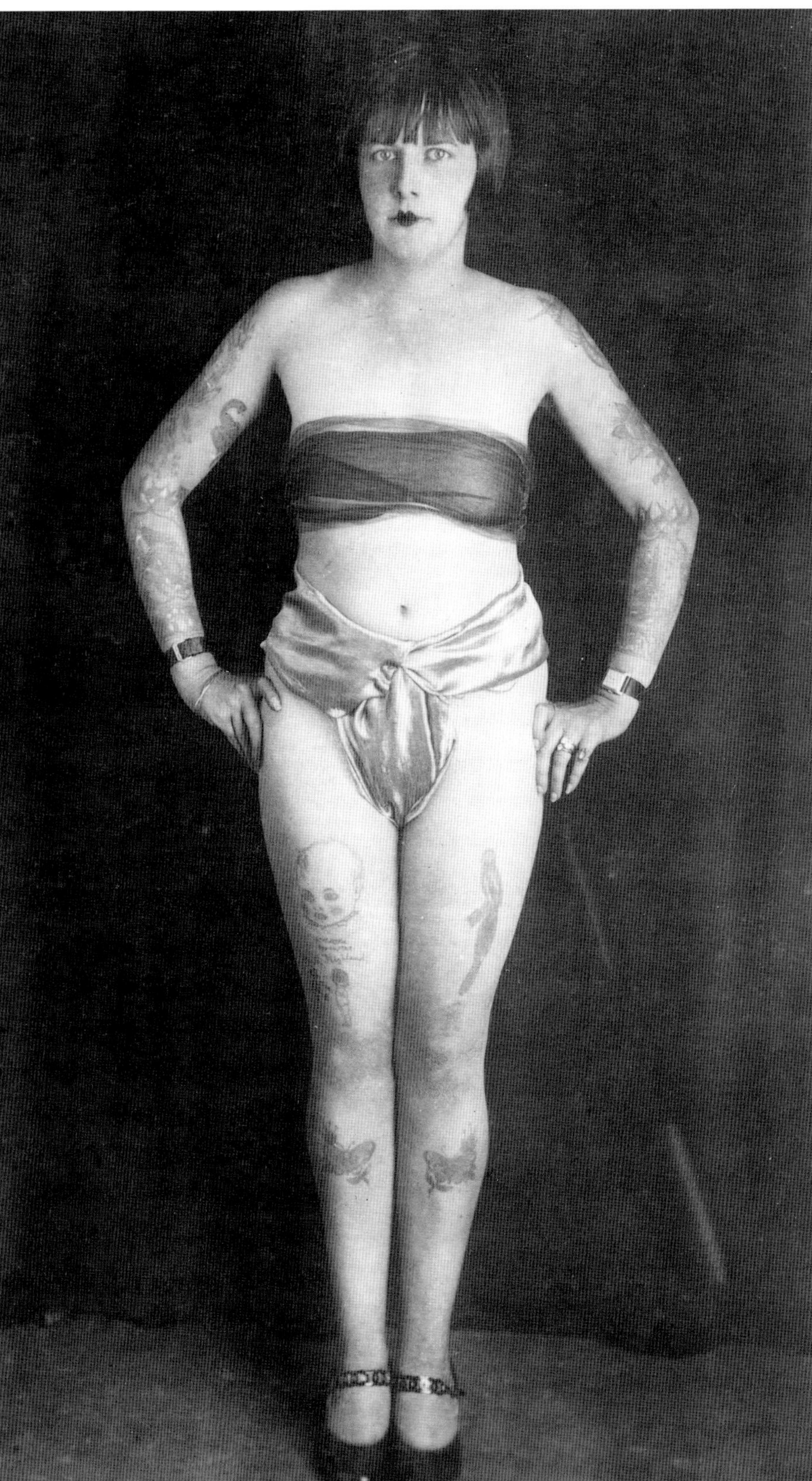

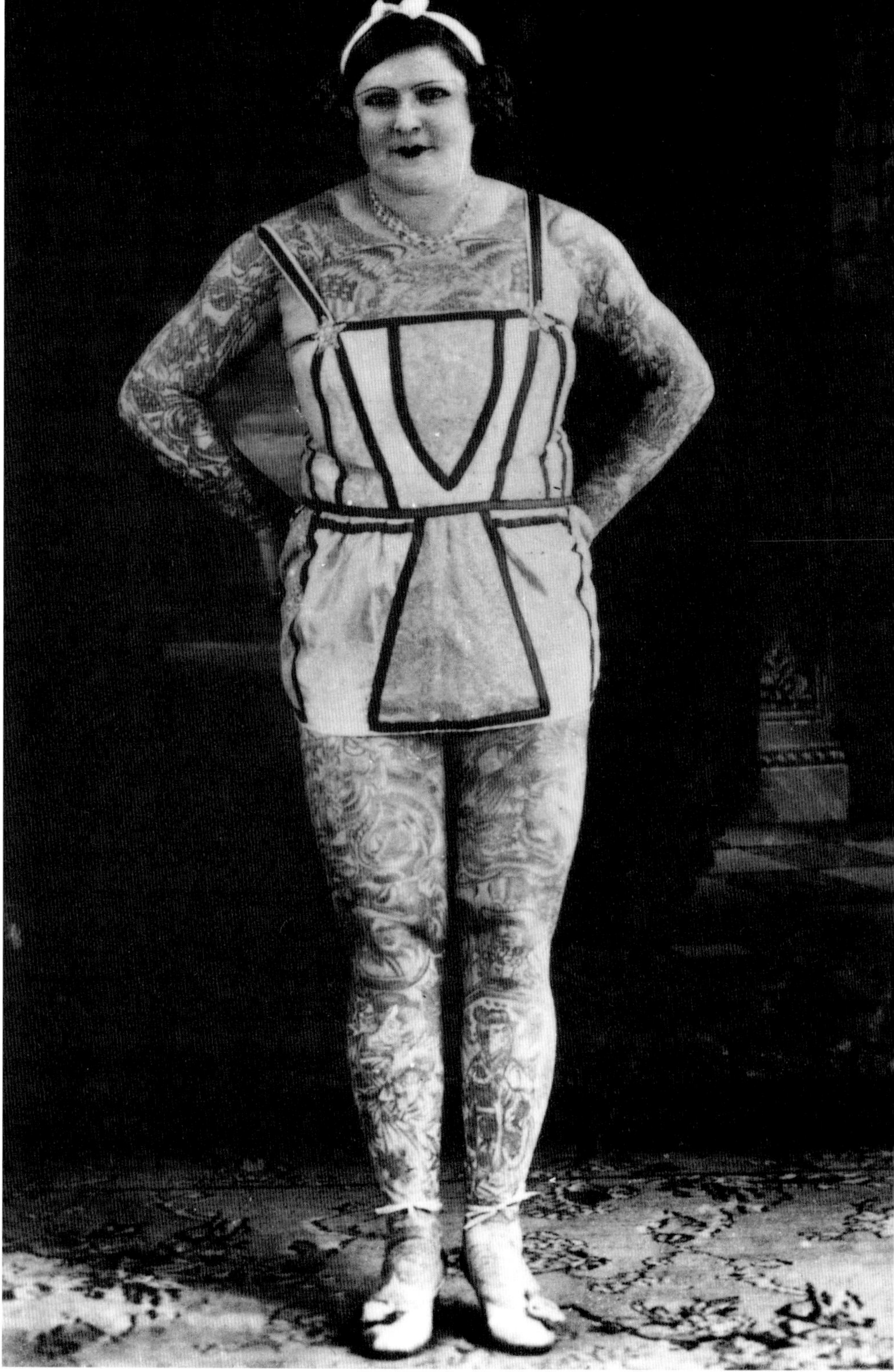

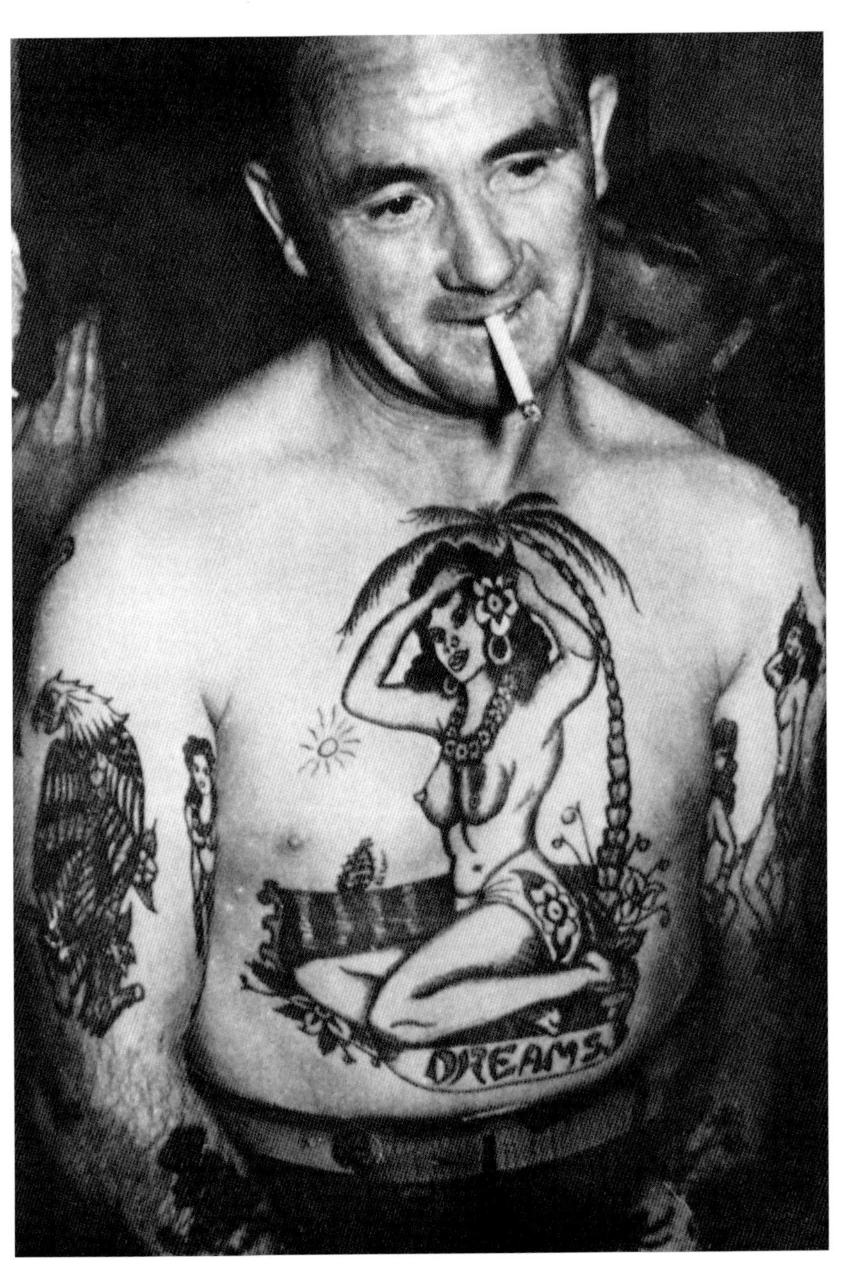

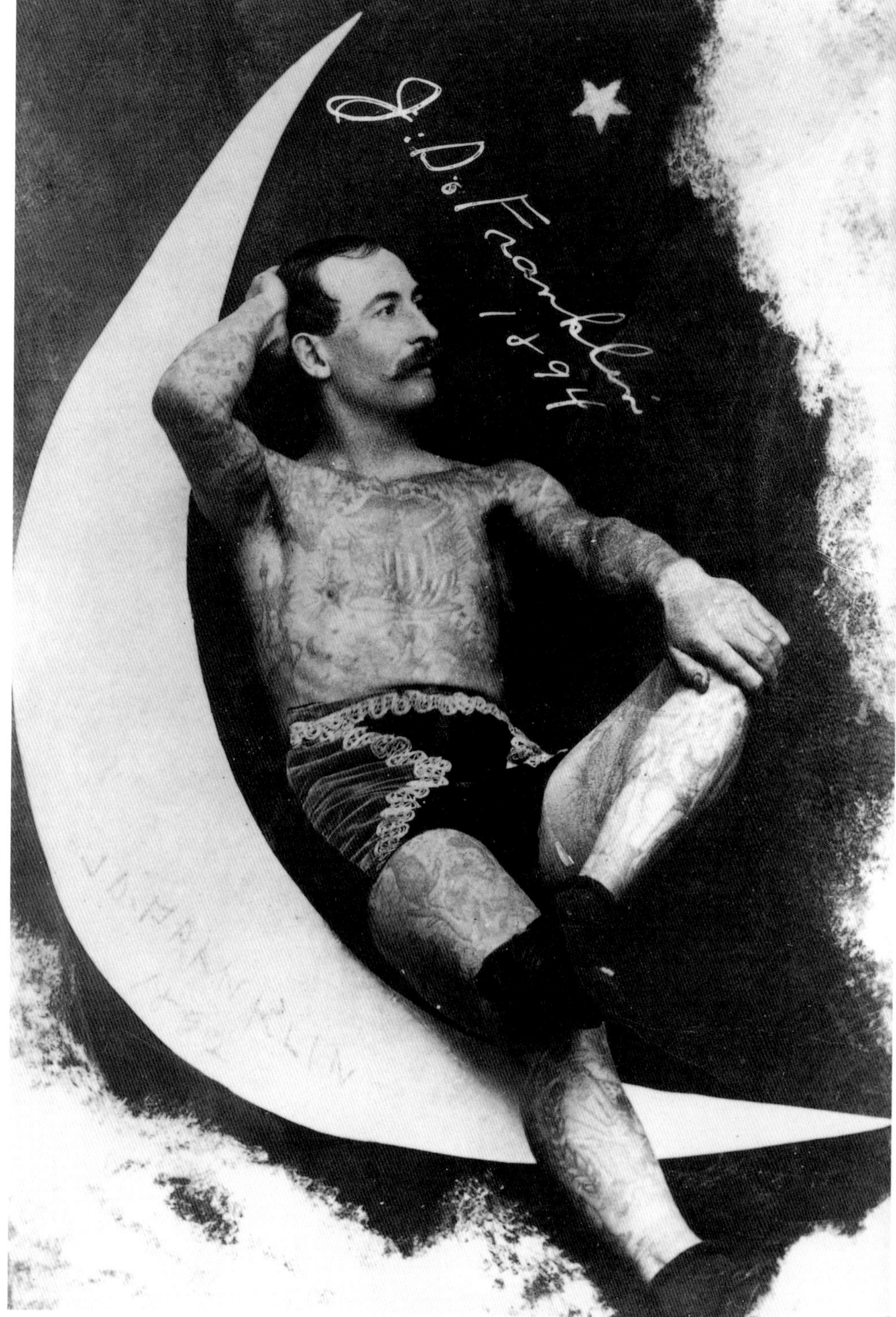

J. D. Franklin
1894

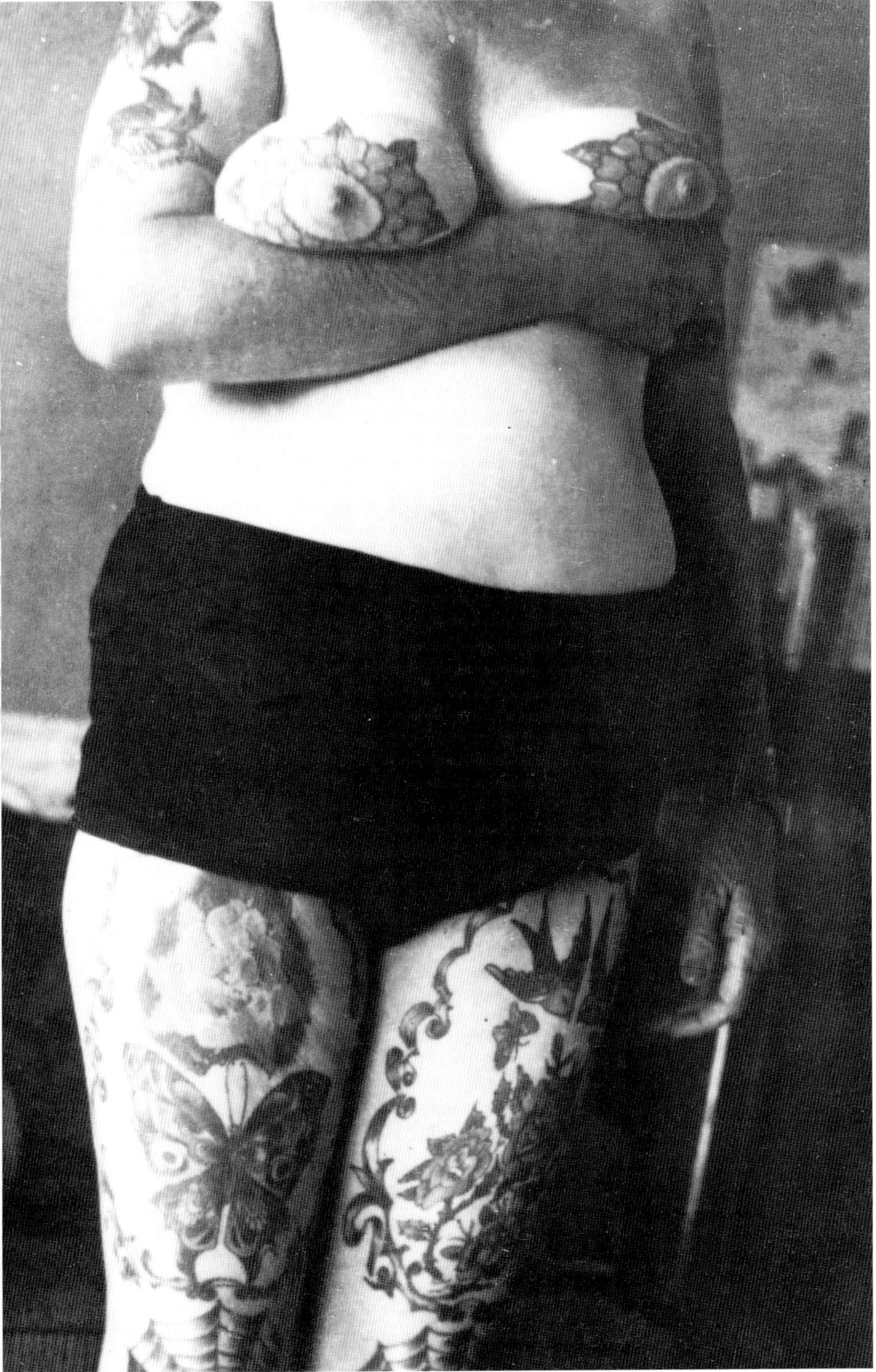

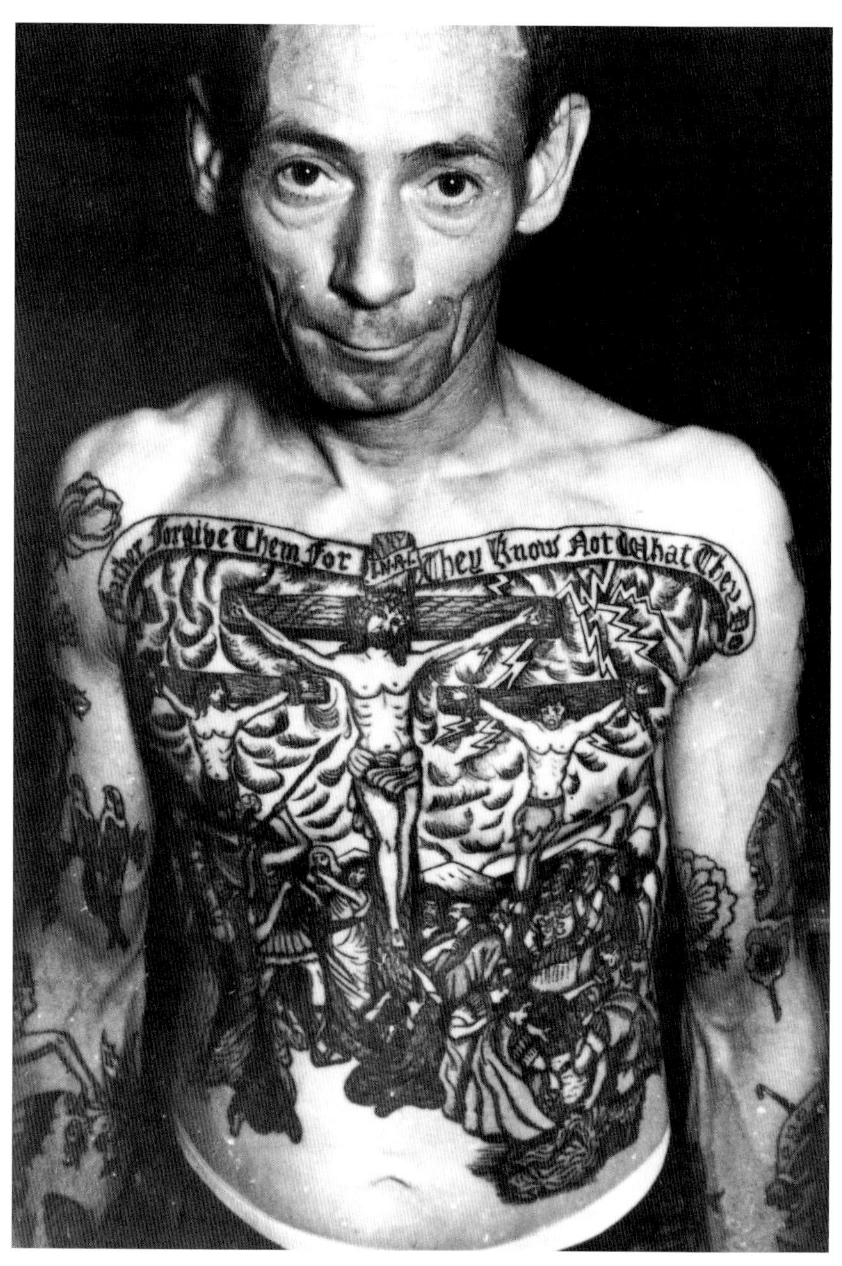
Father Forgive Them For They Know Not What They Do
INRI

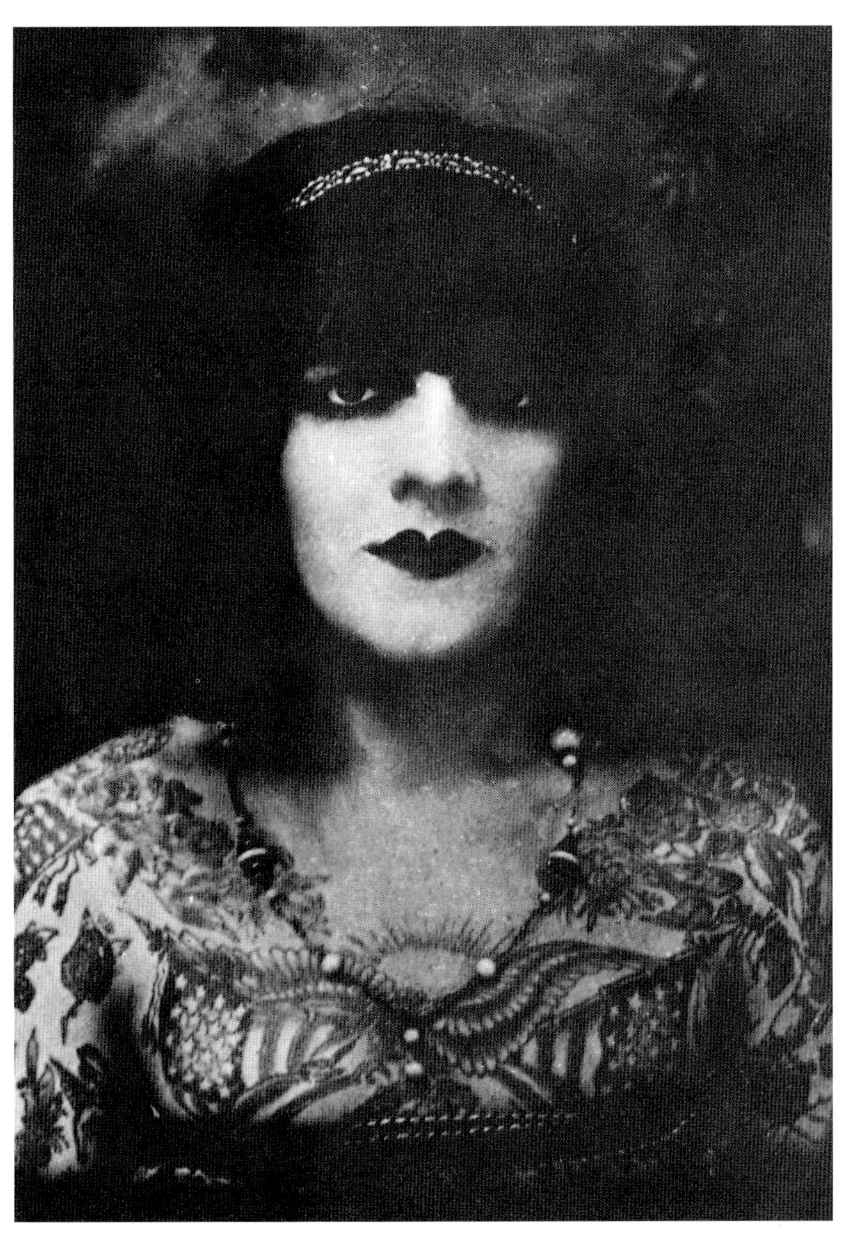

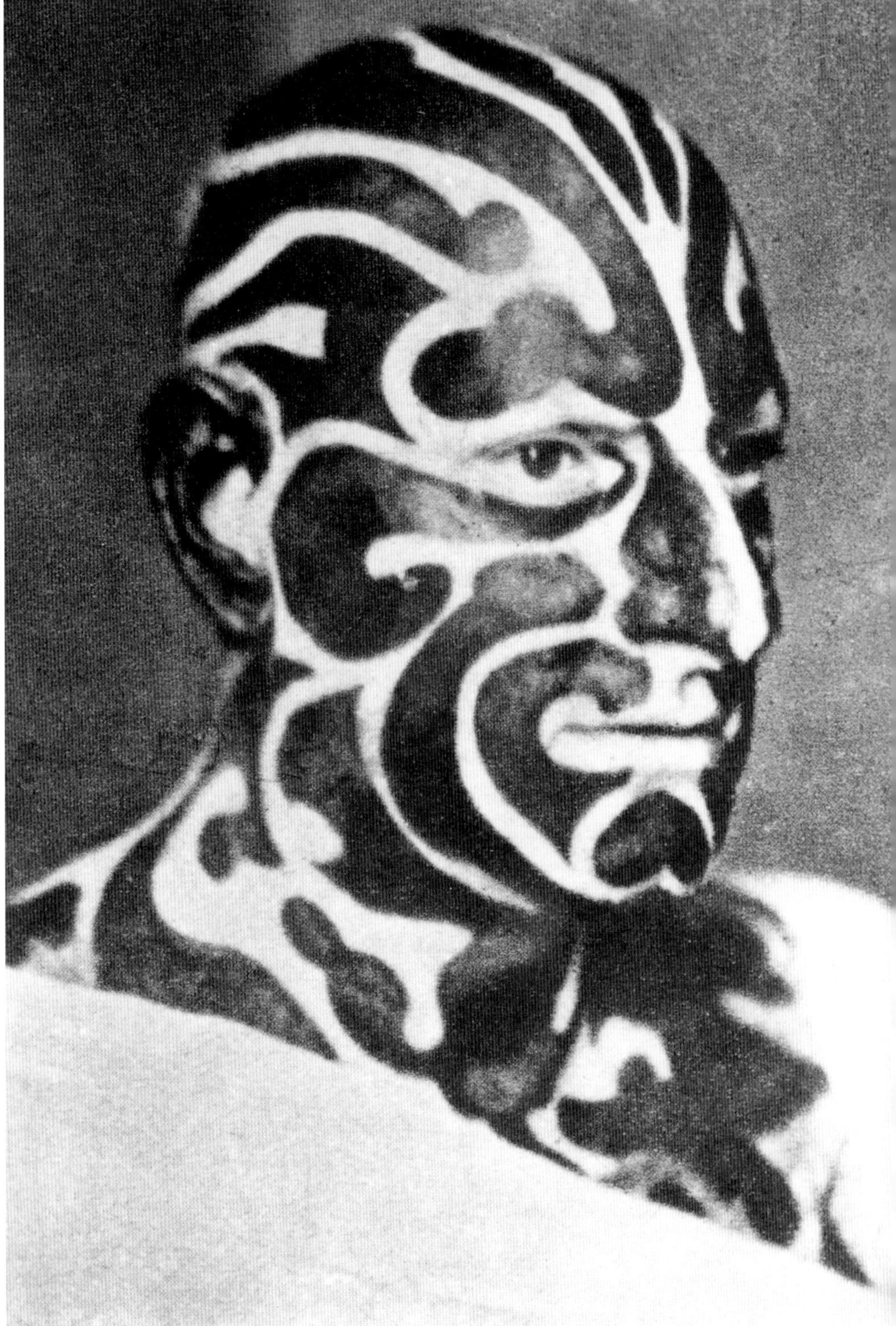

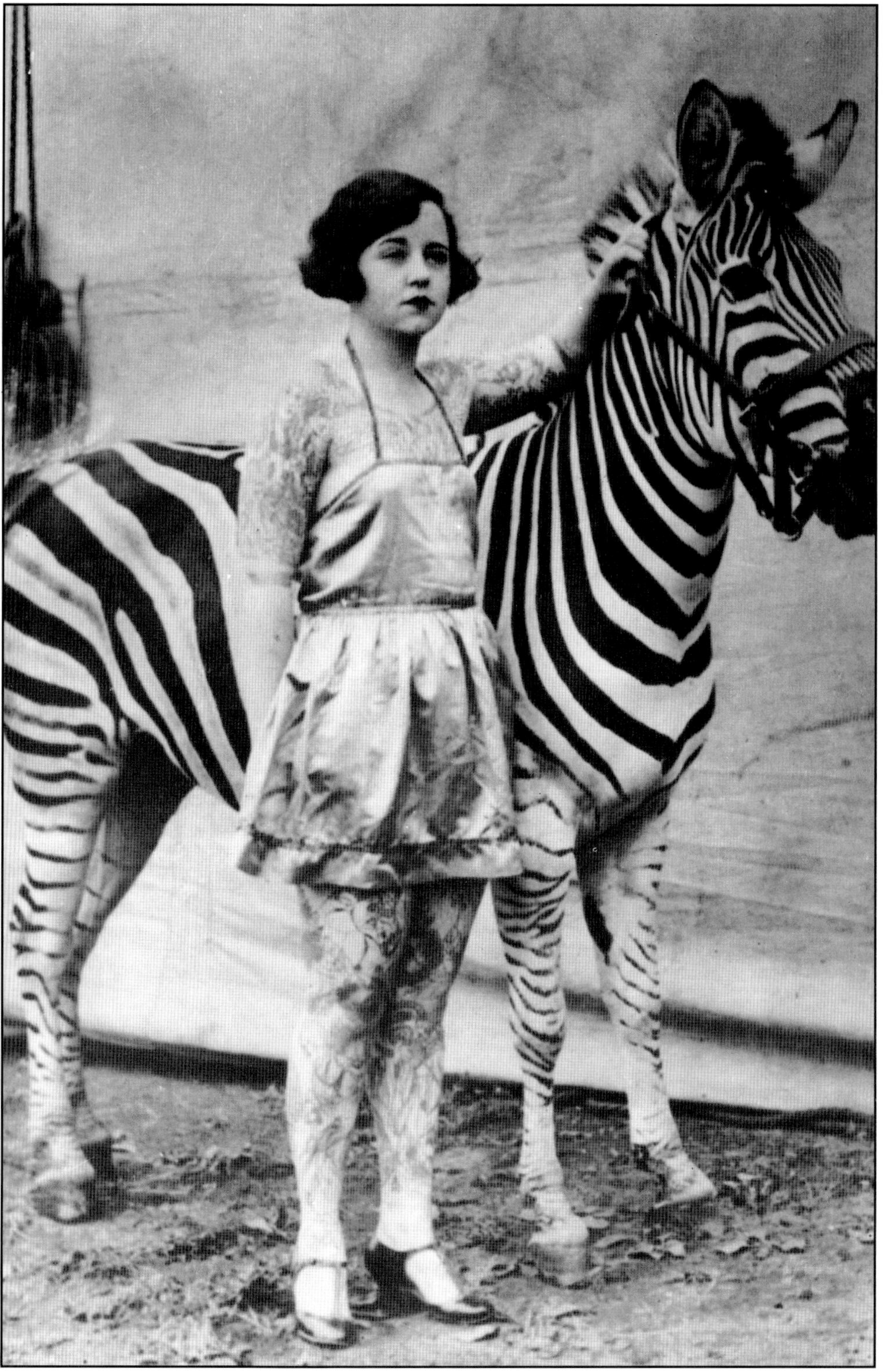

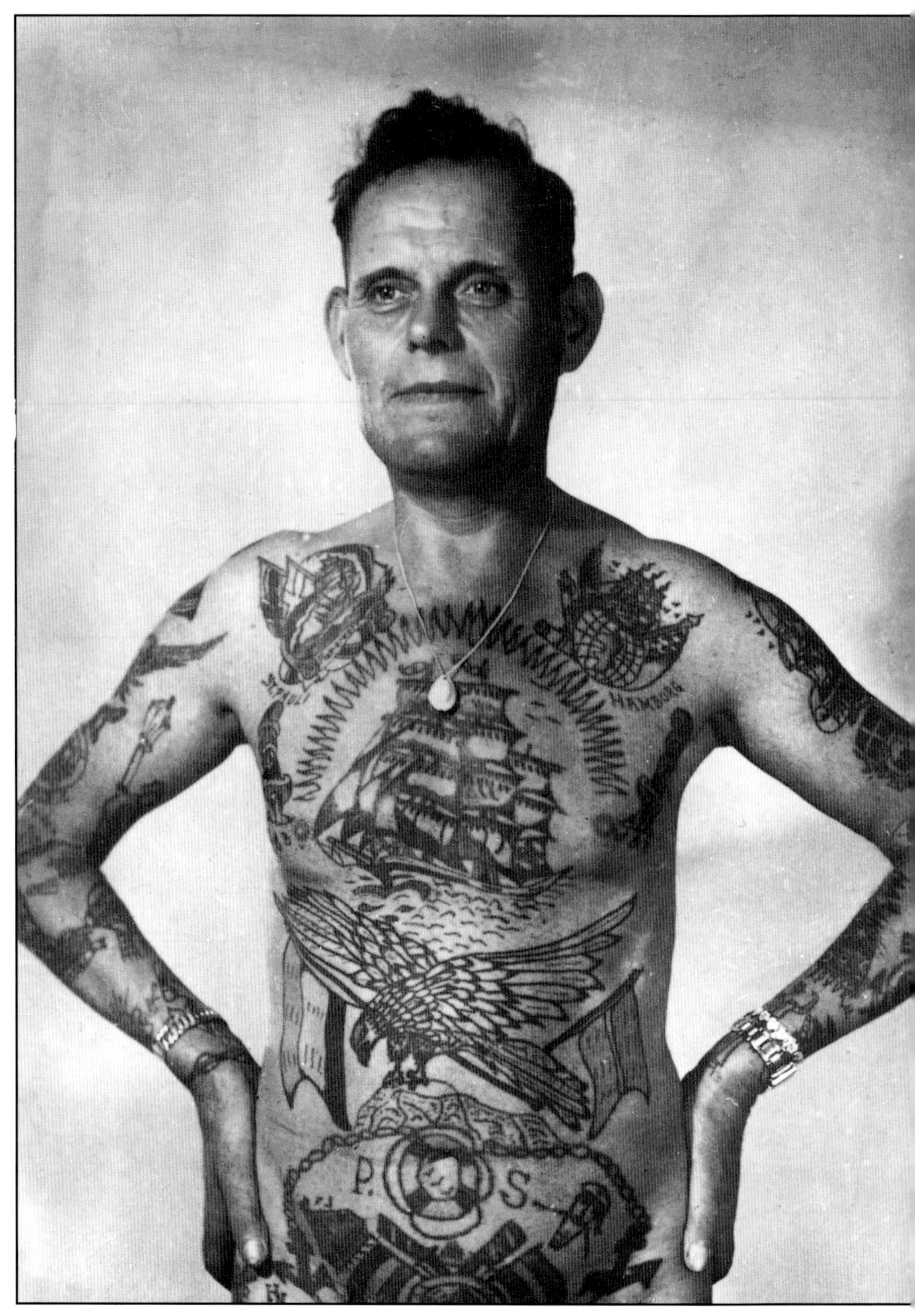

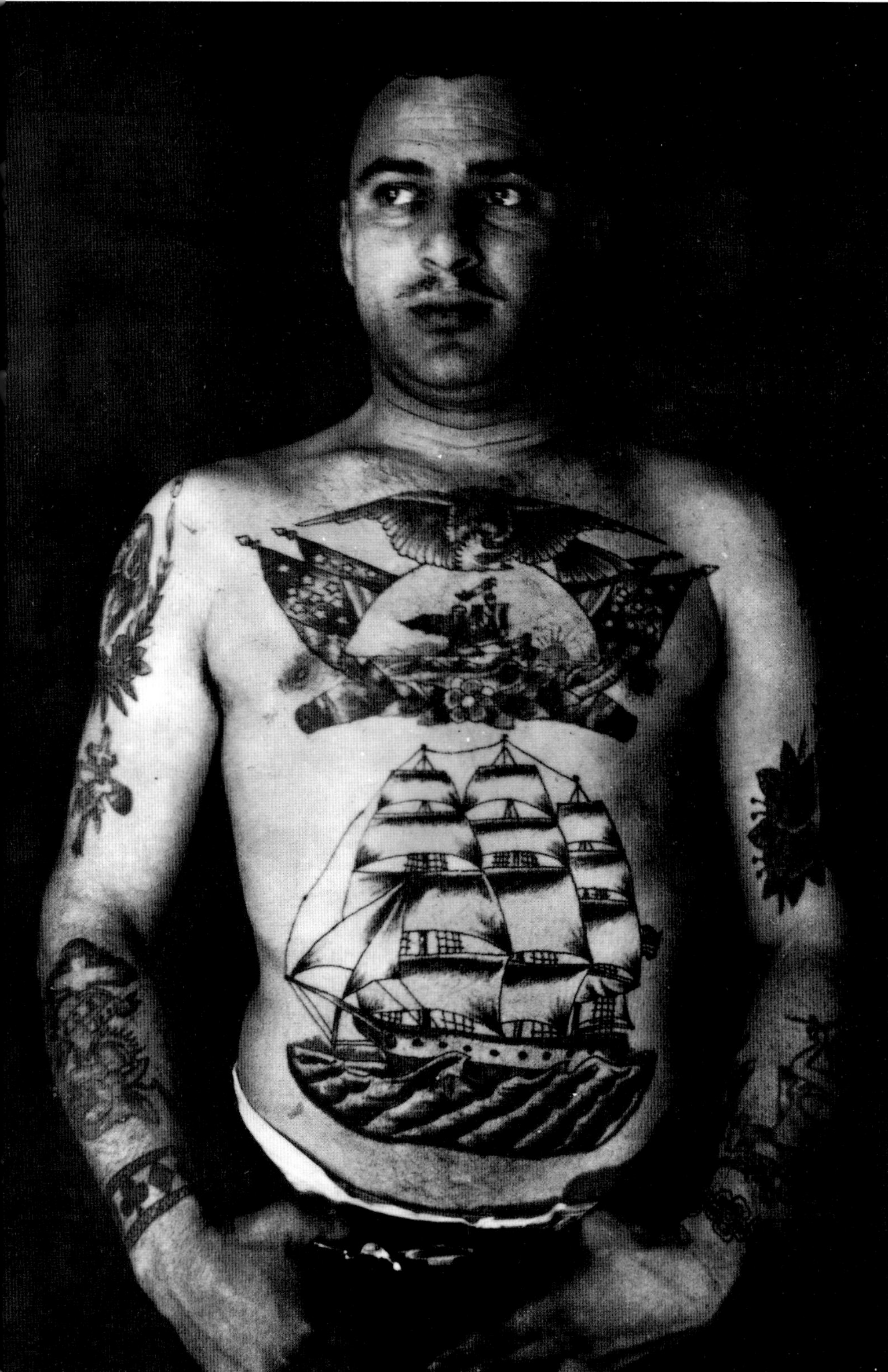

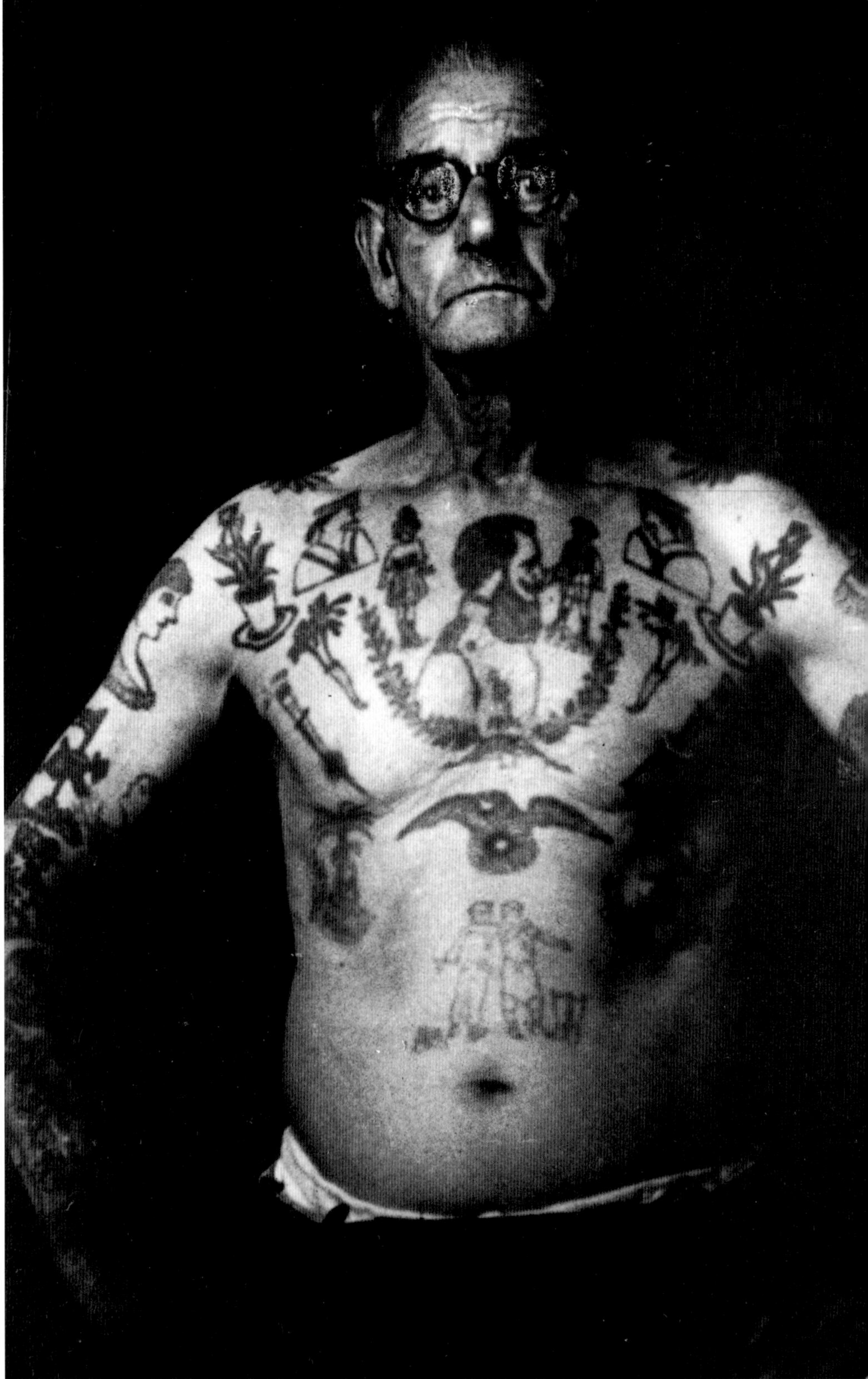

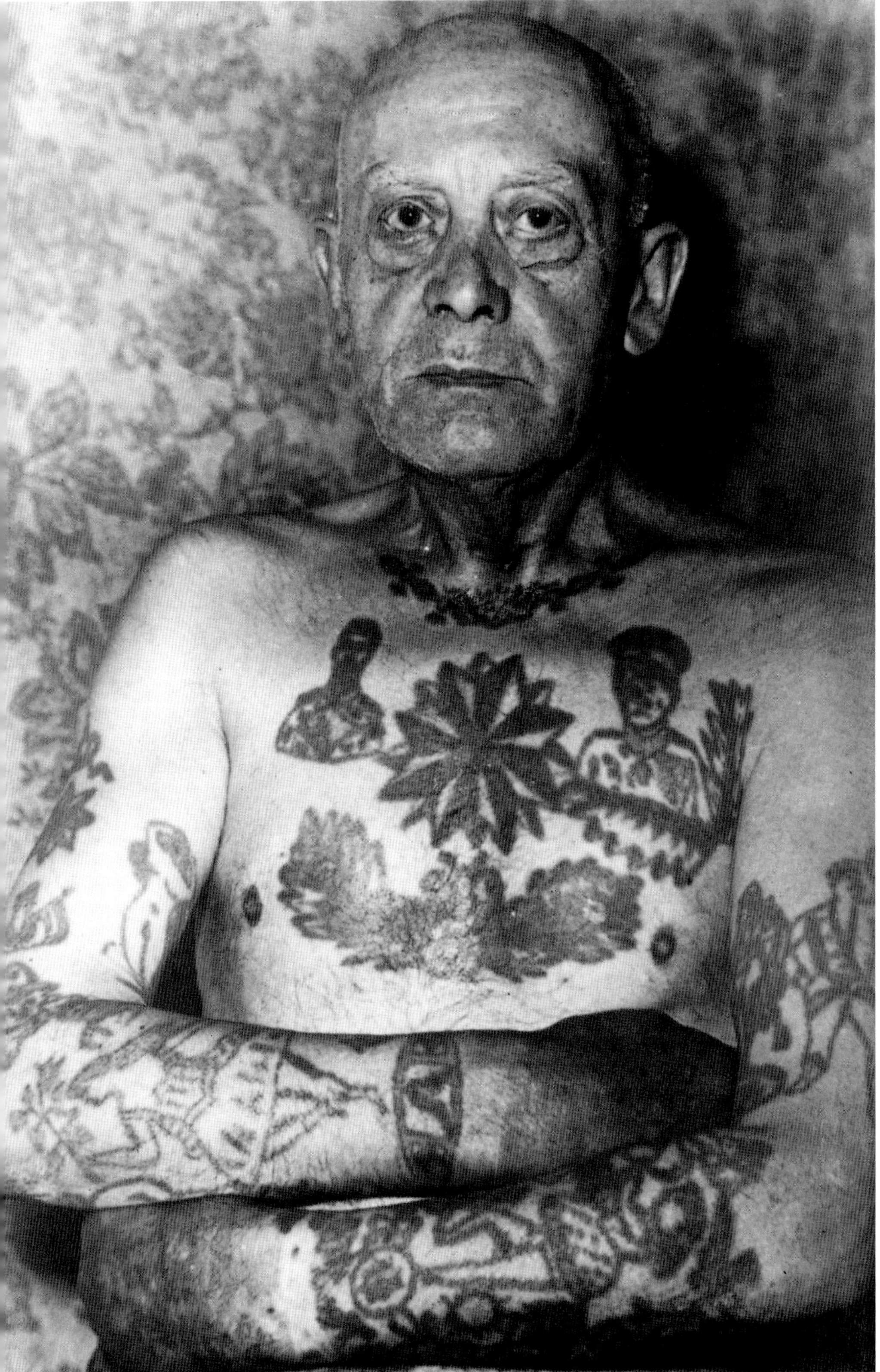

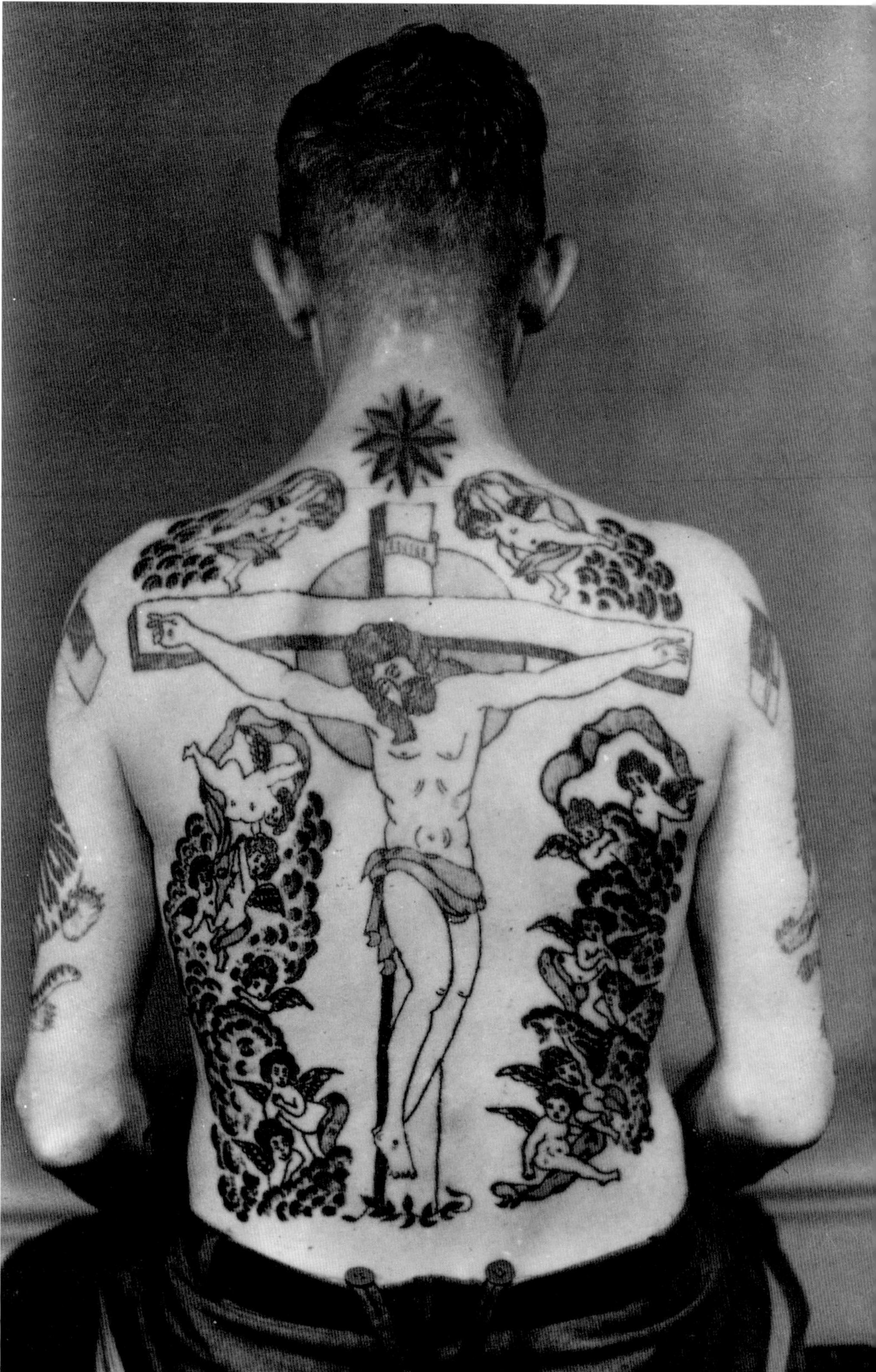

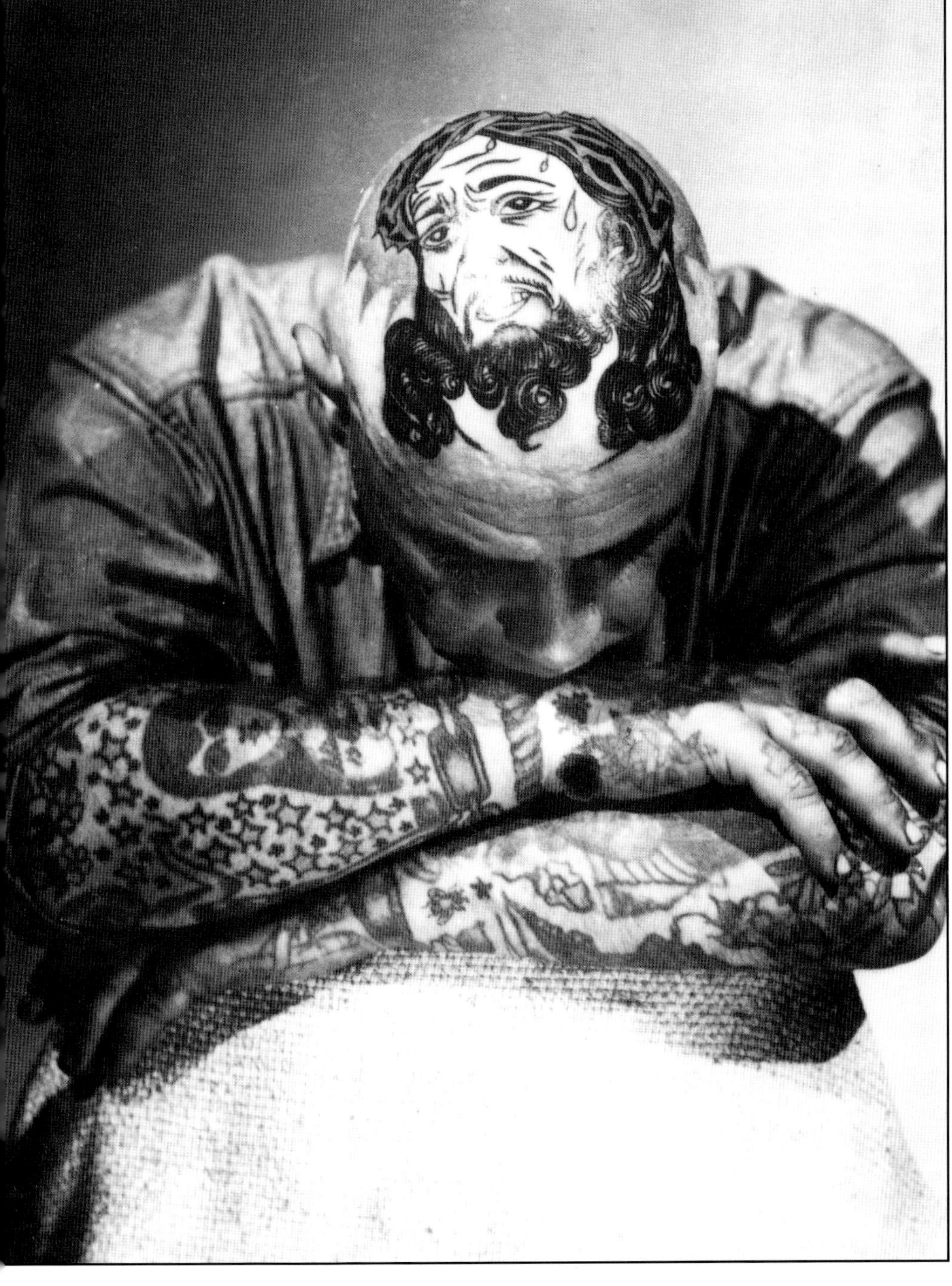

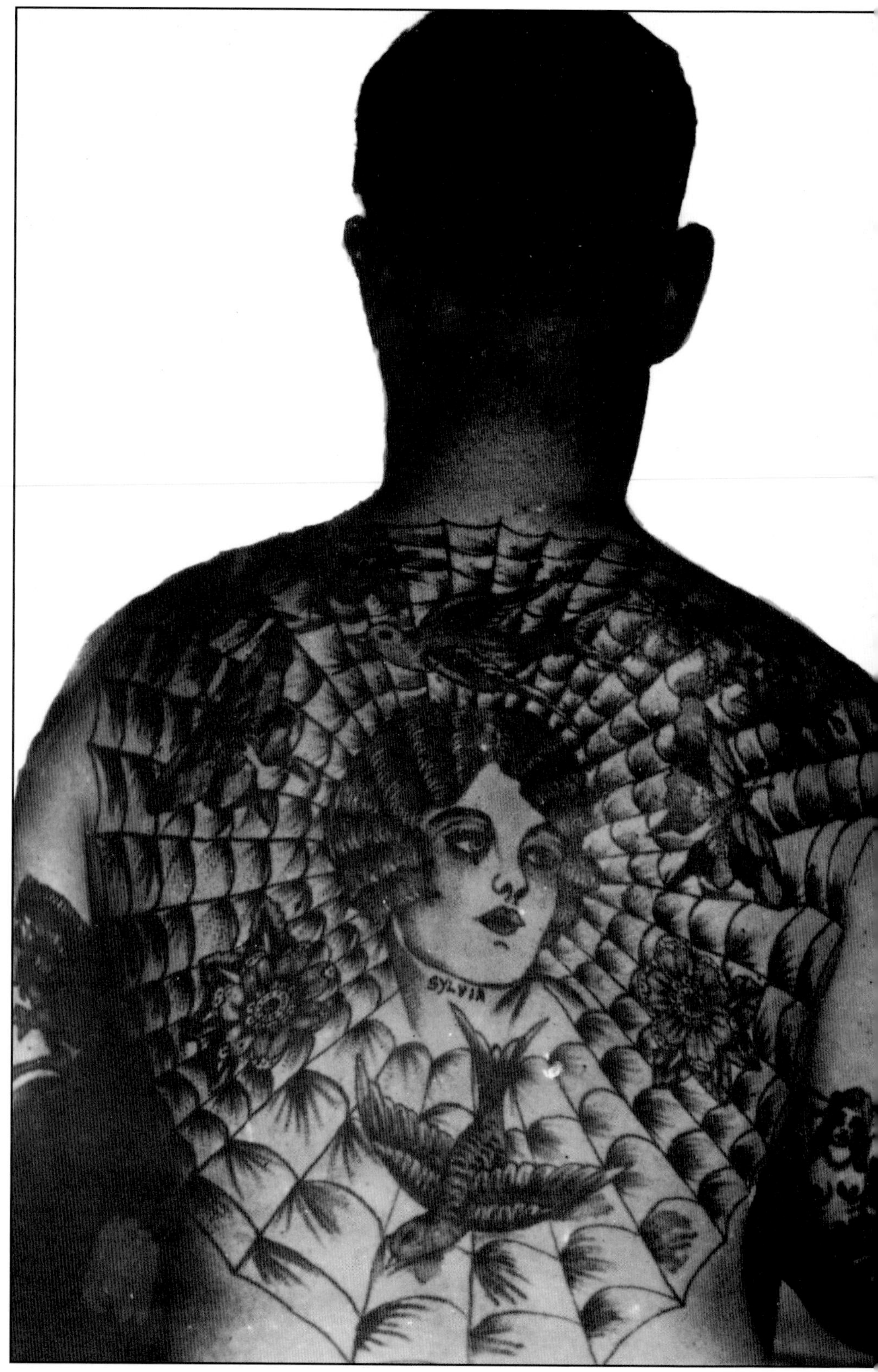
SYLVIA

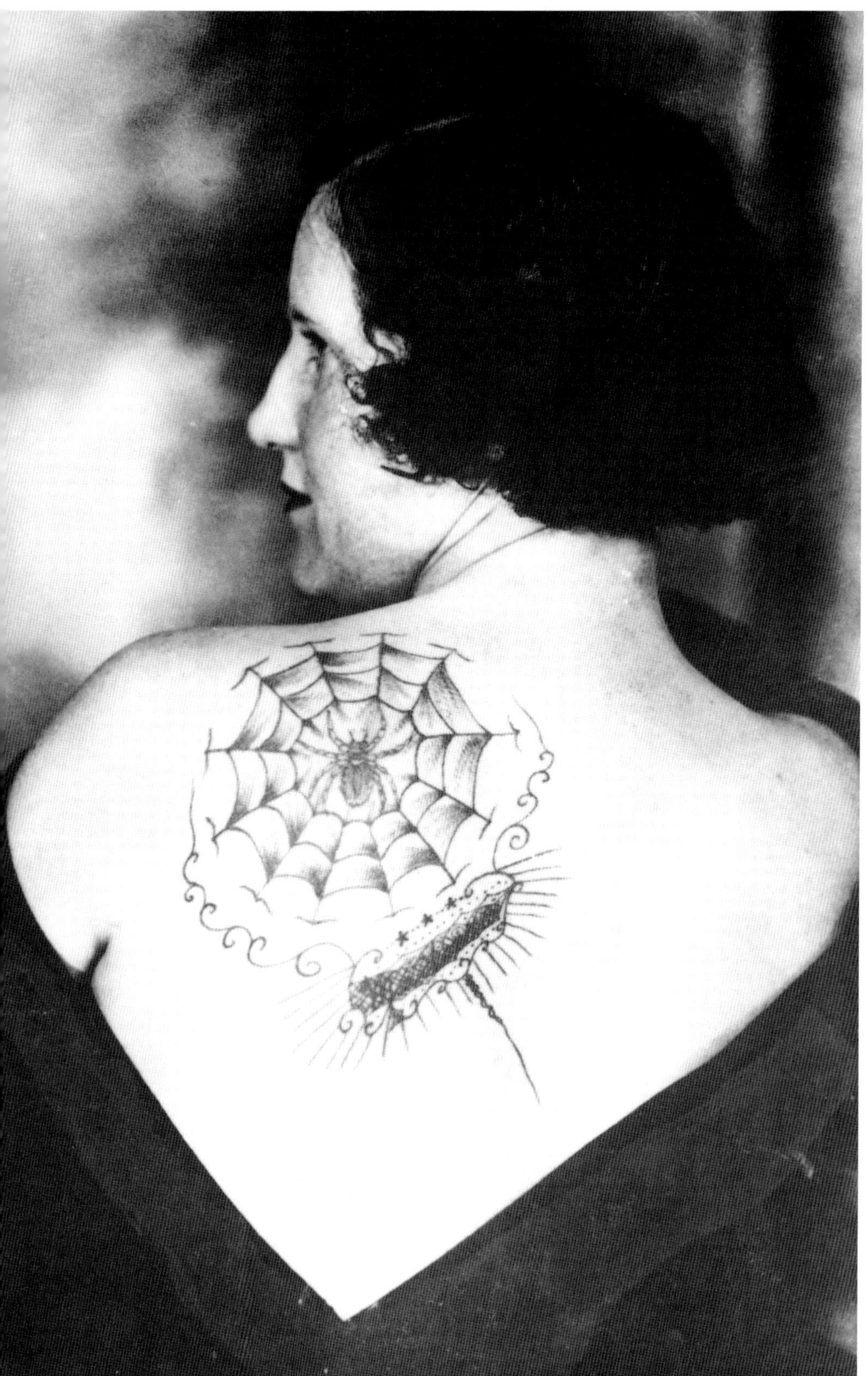

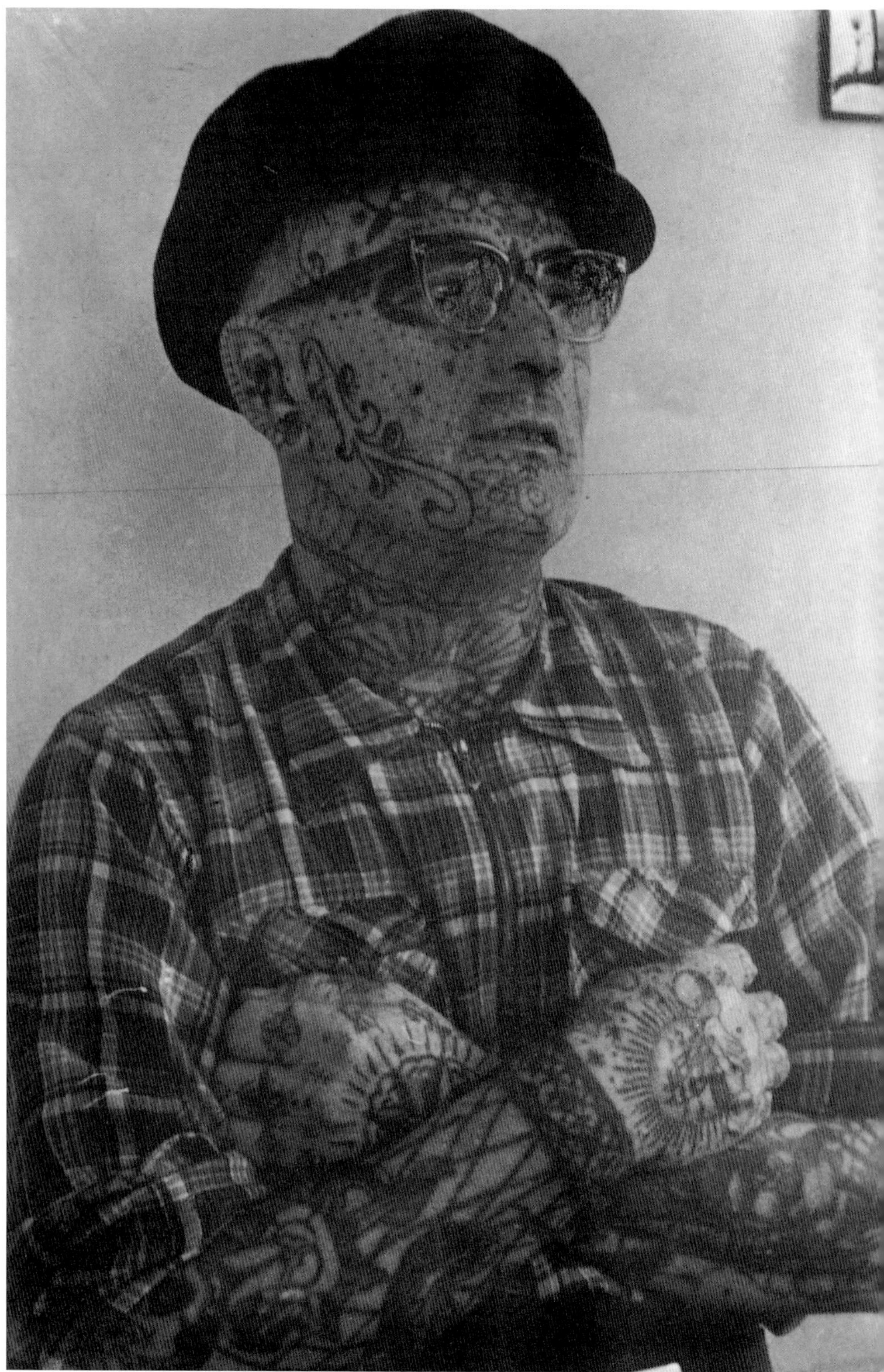

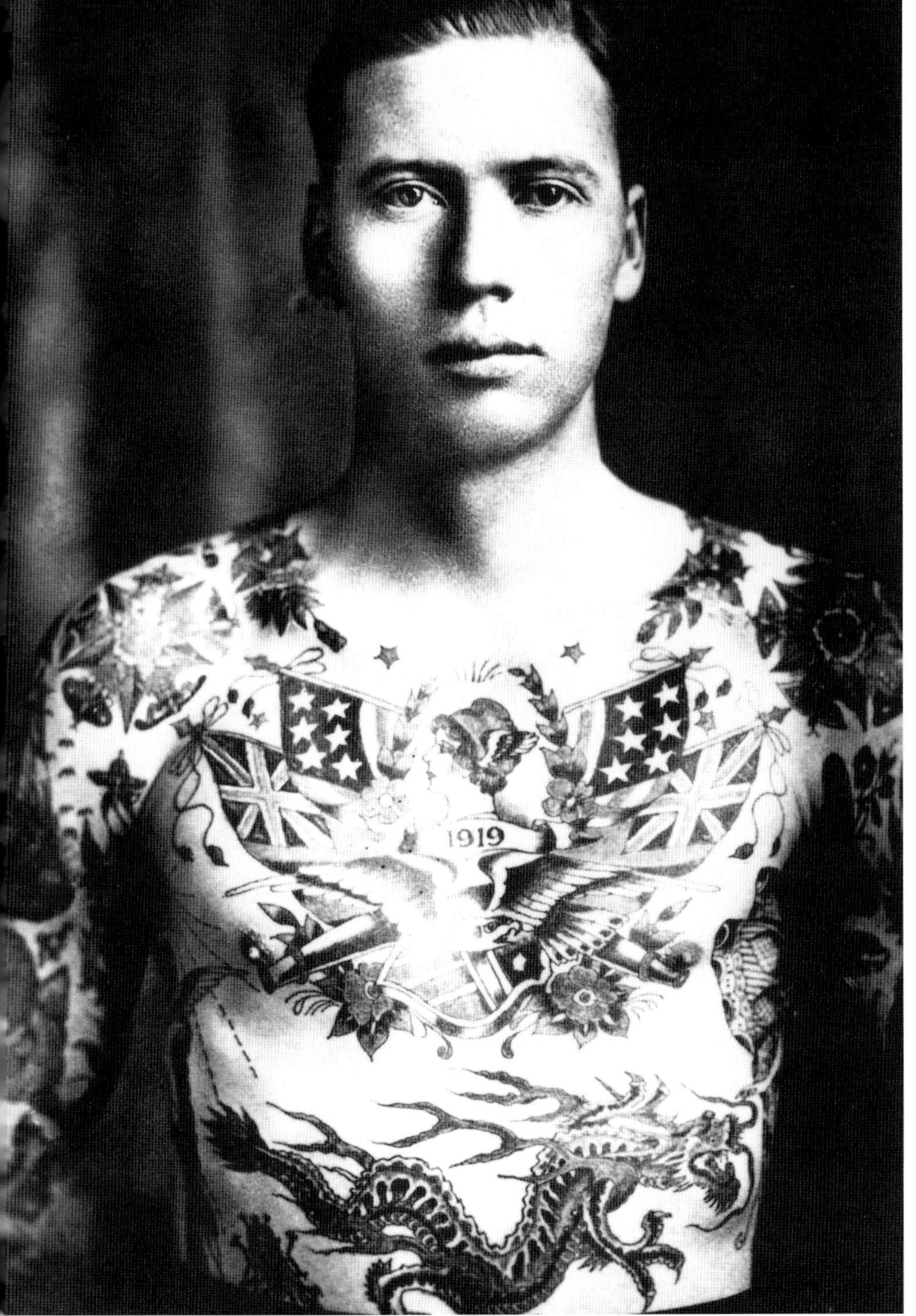

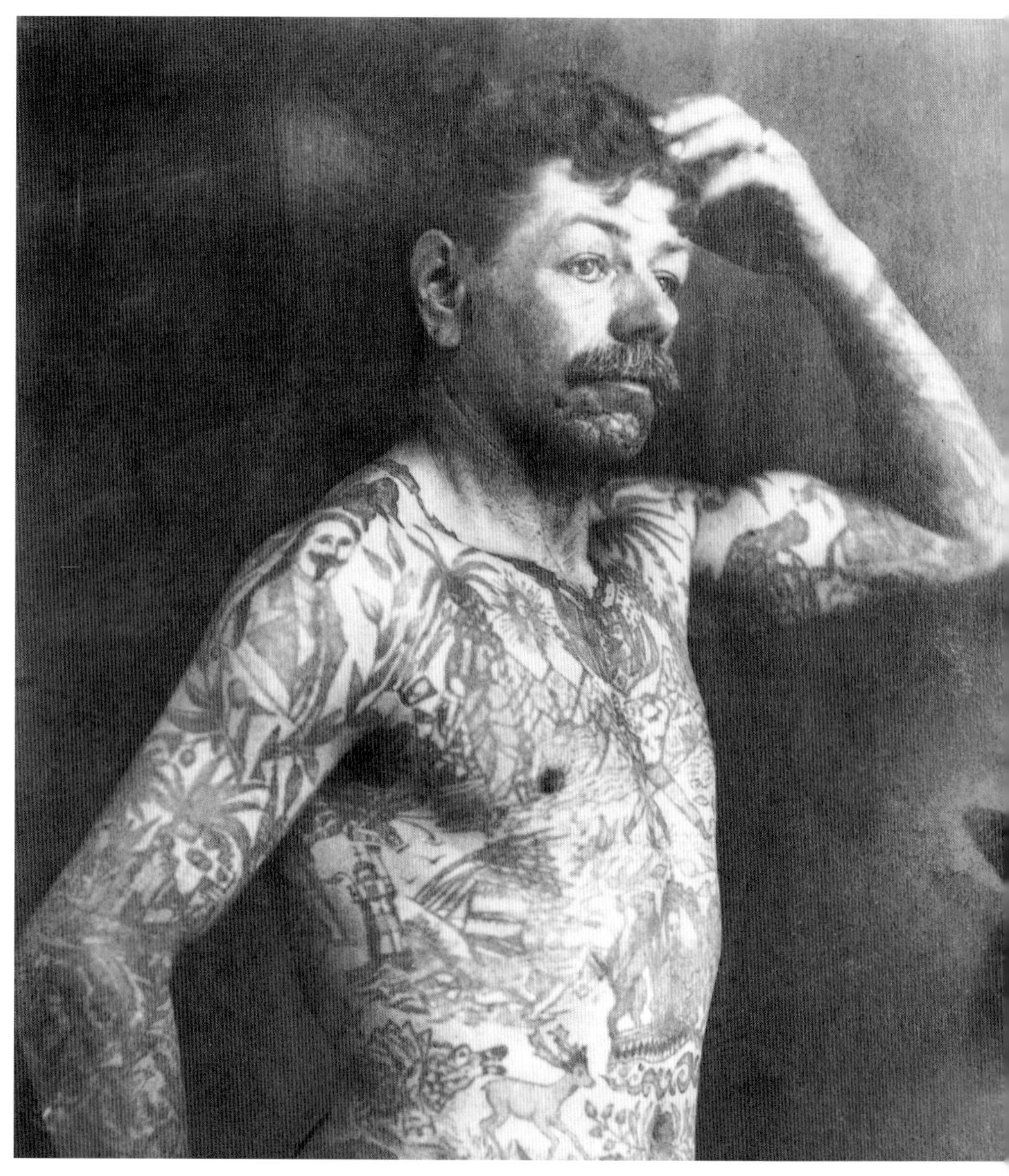

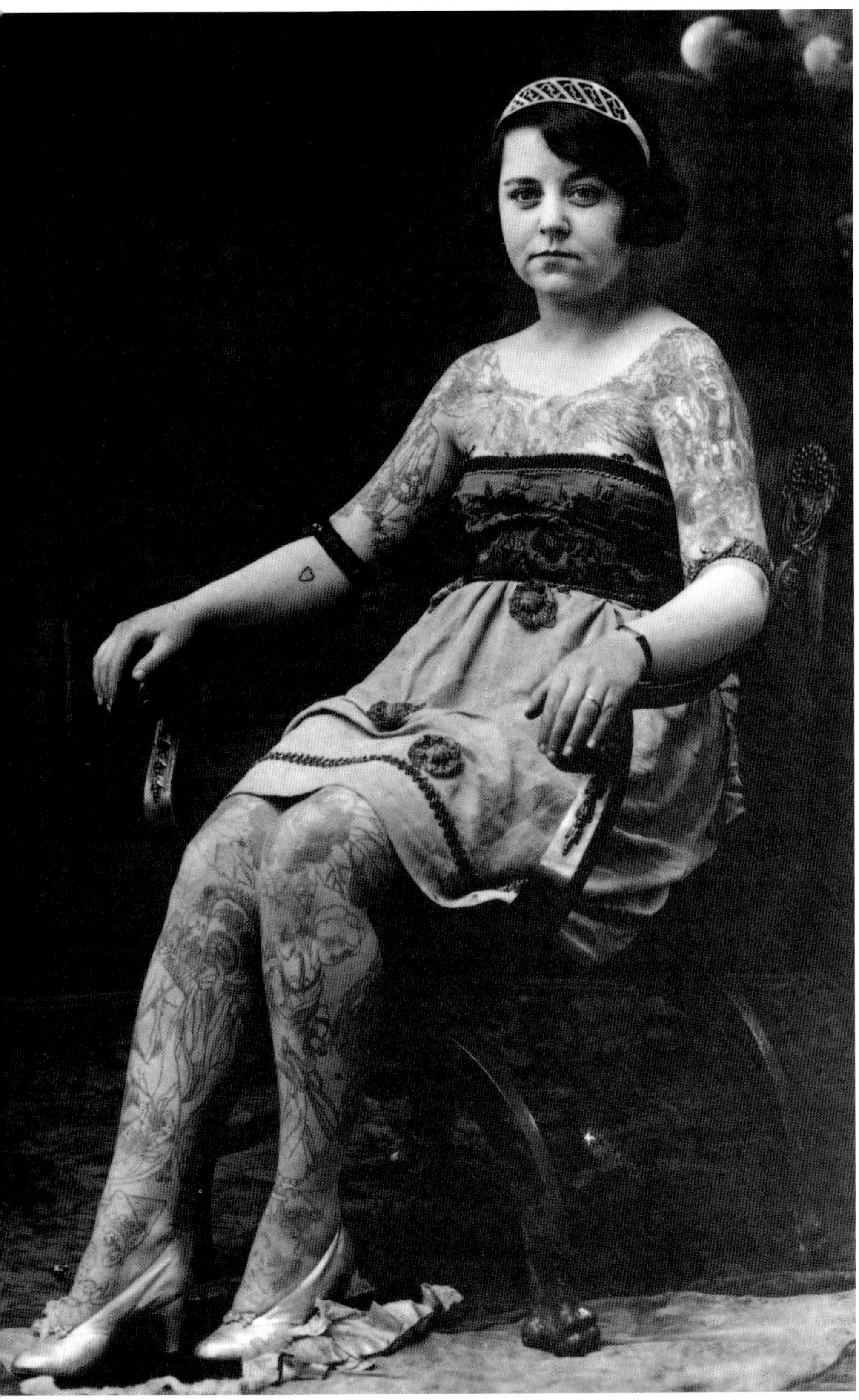

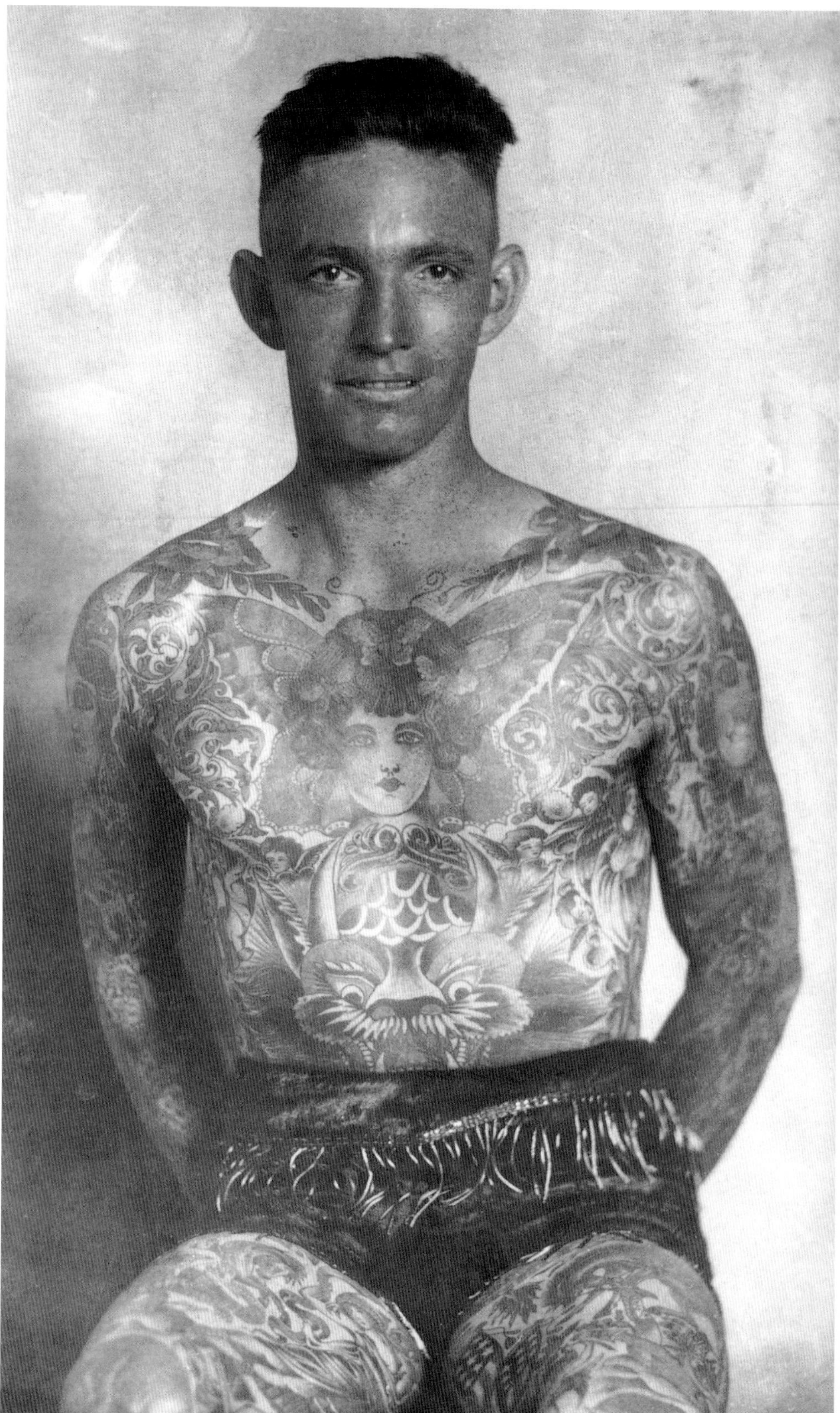

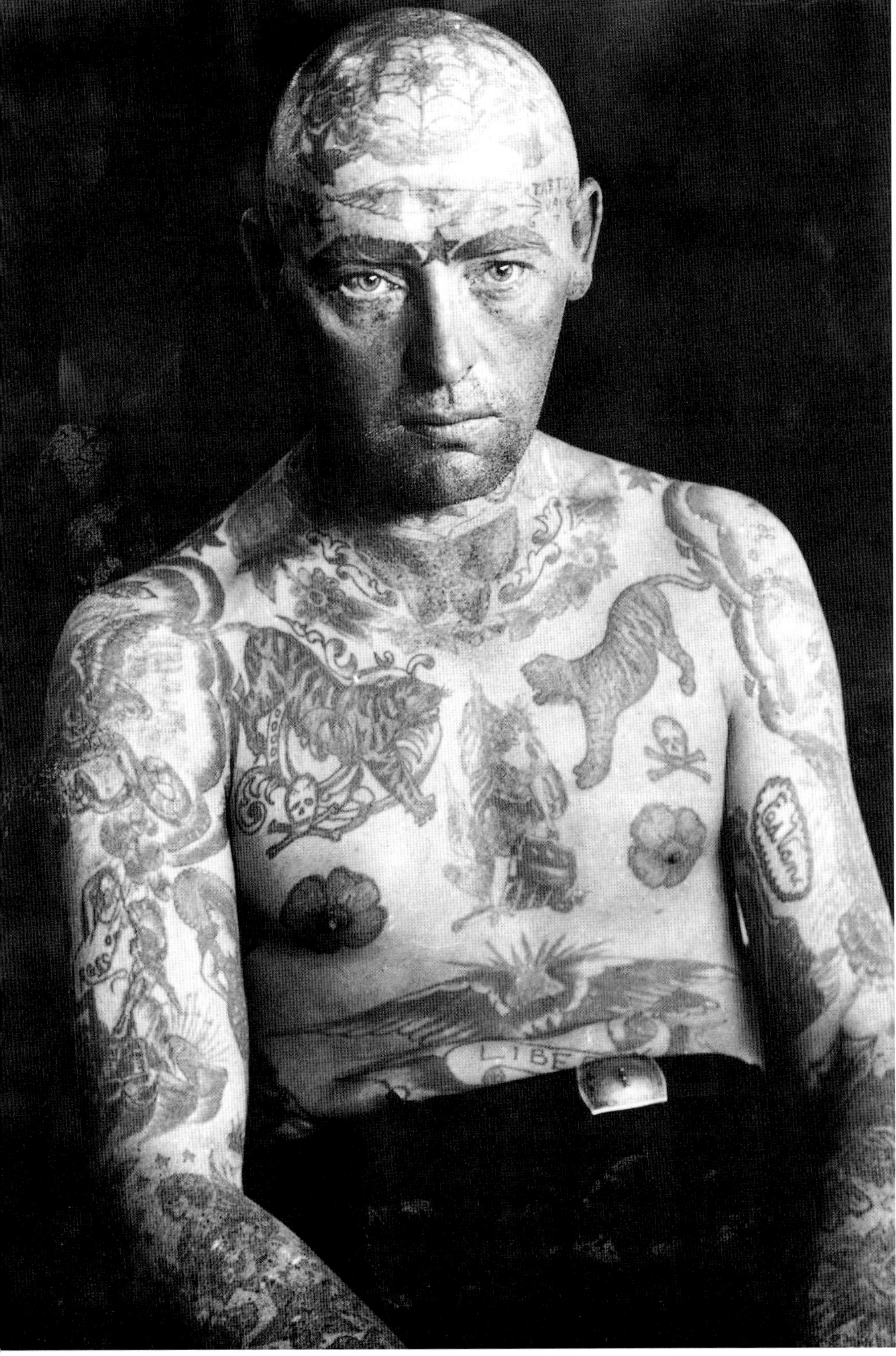

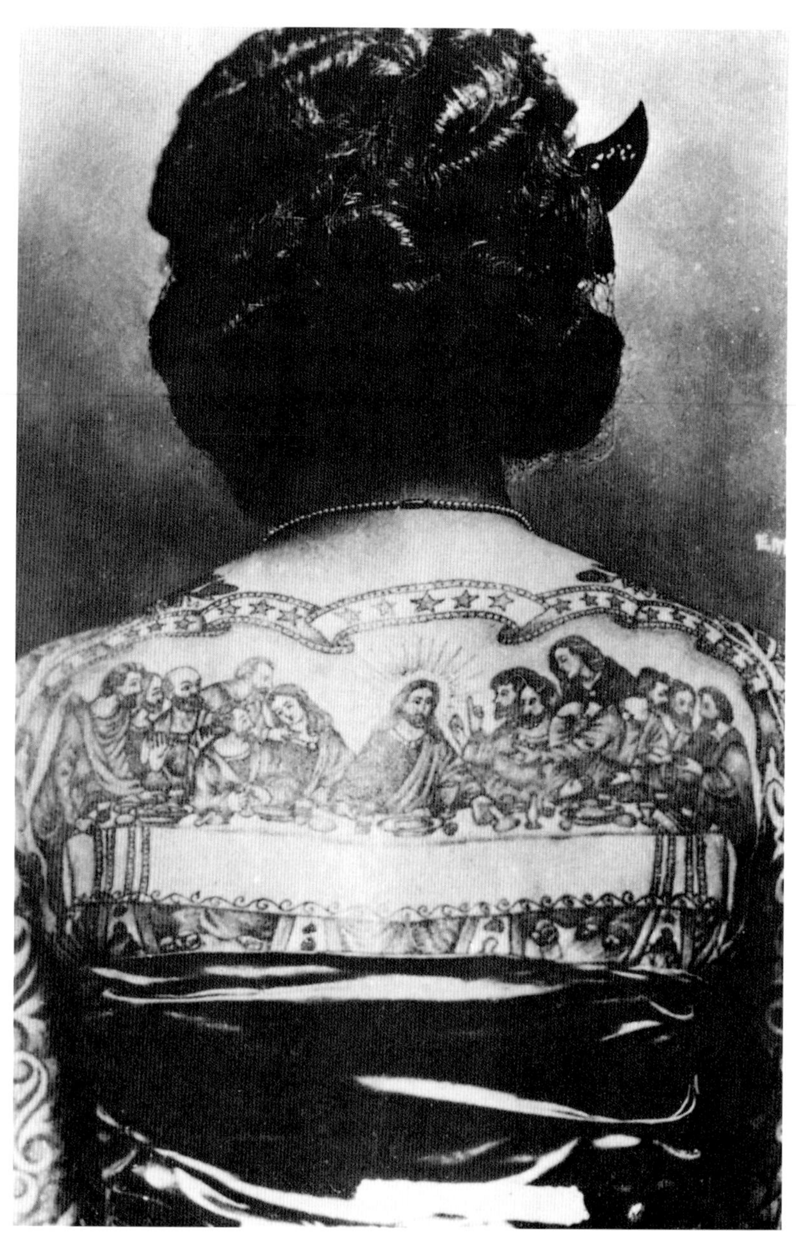

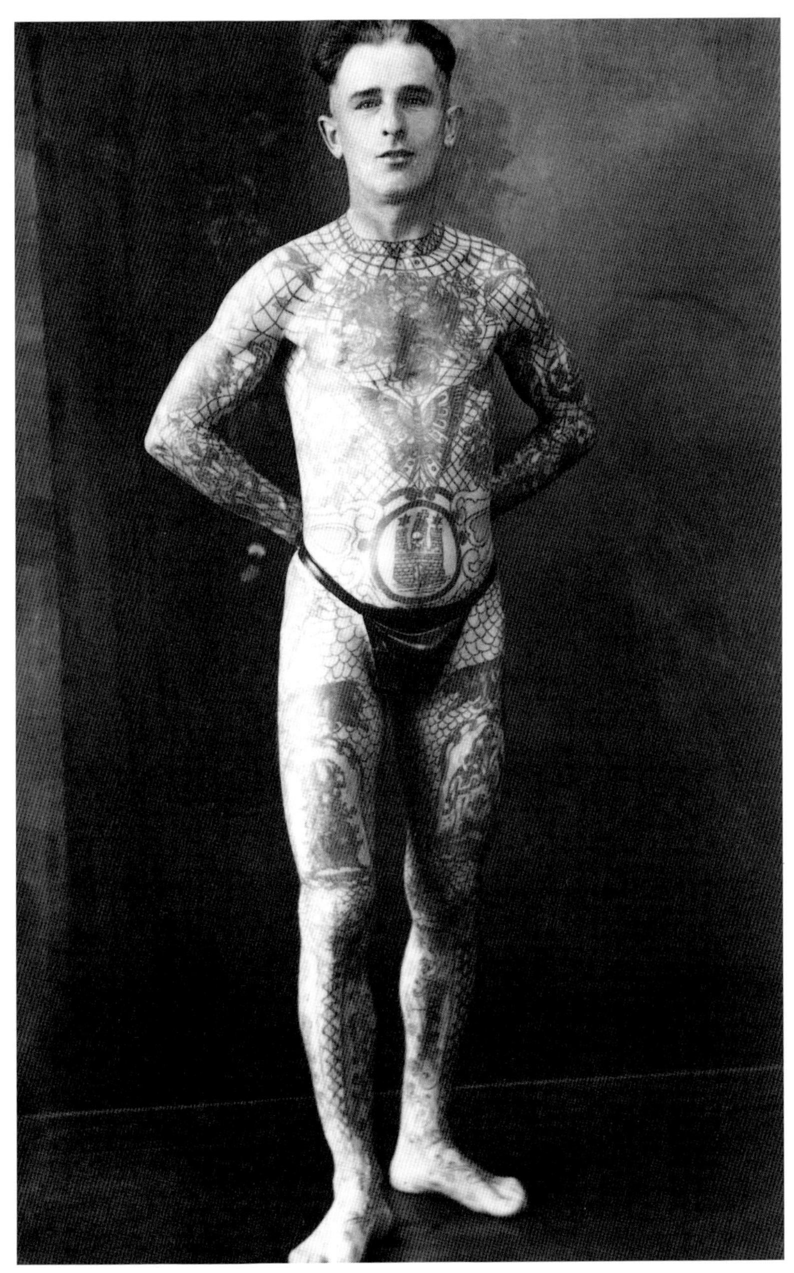

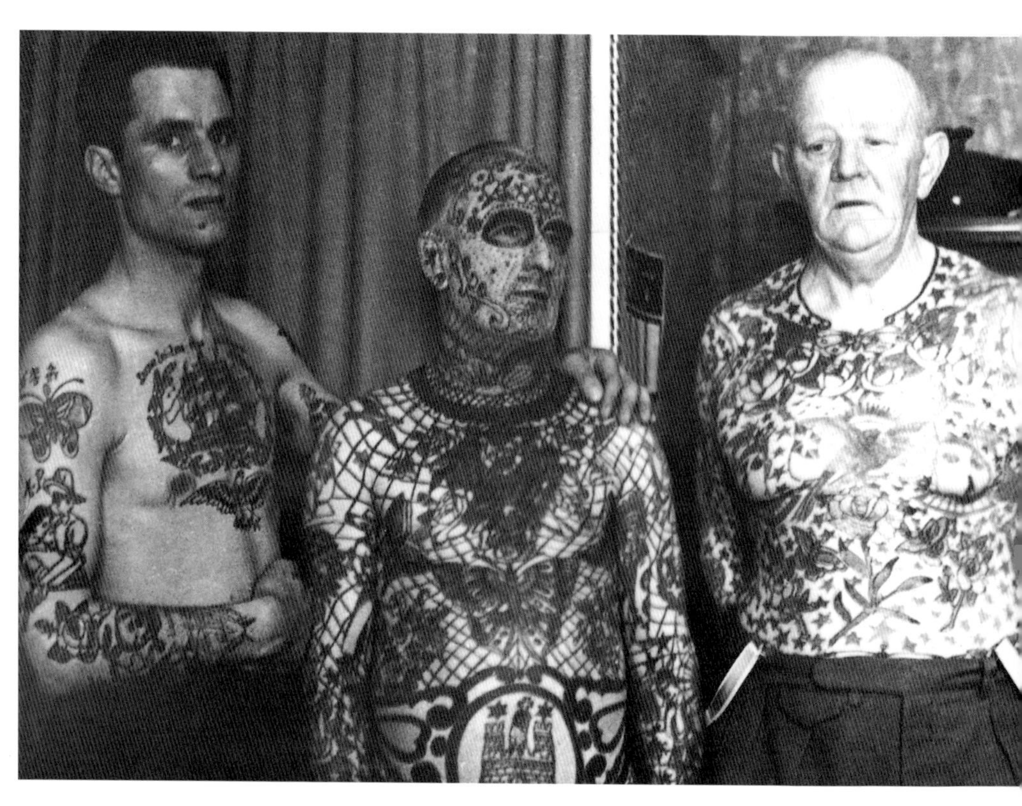

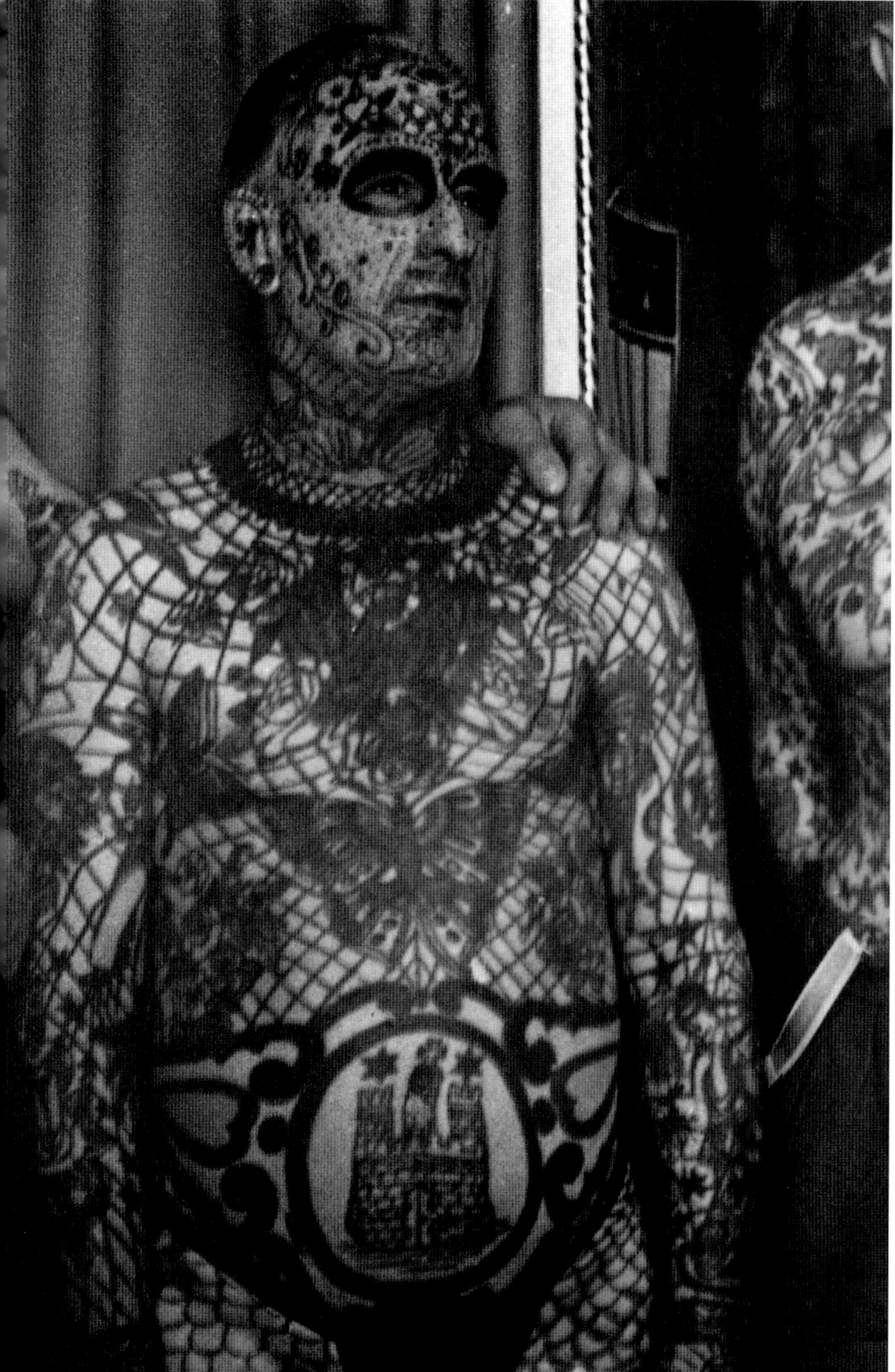

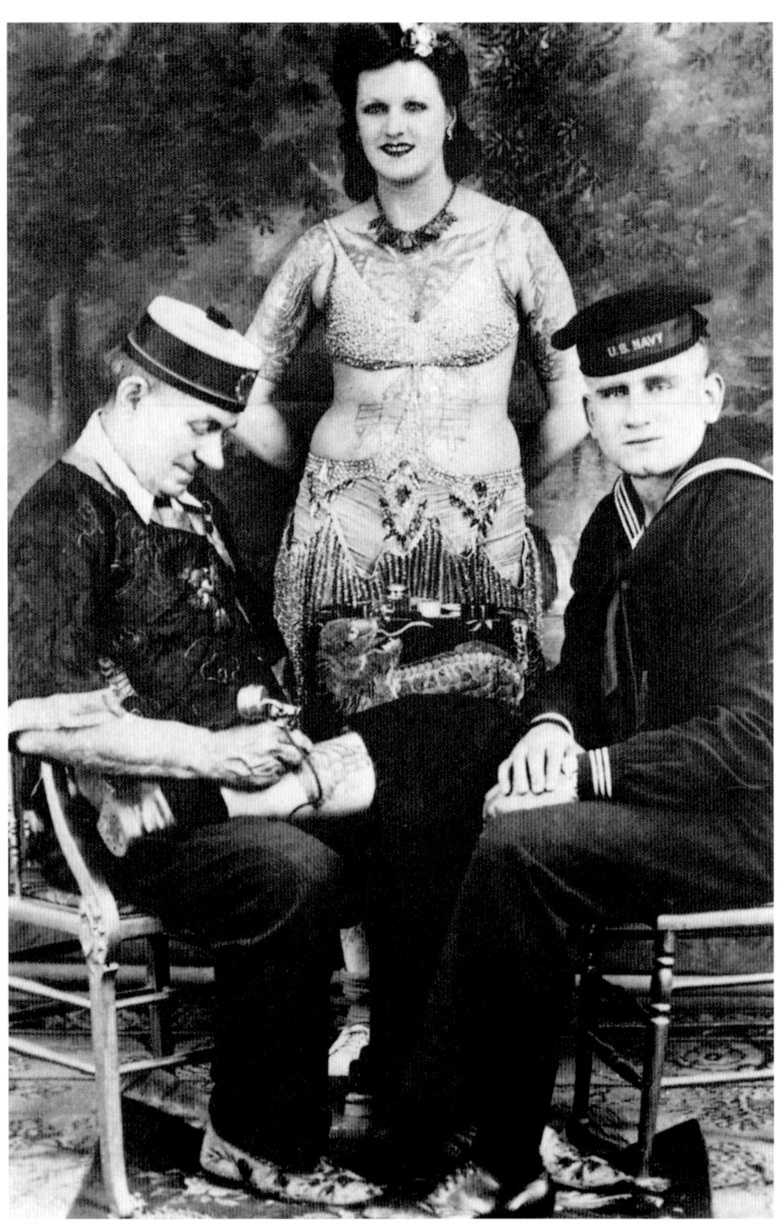
U.S. NAVY

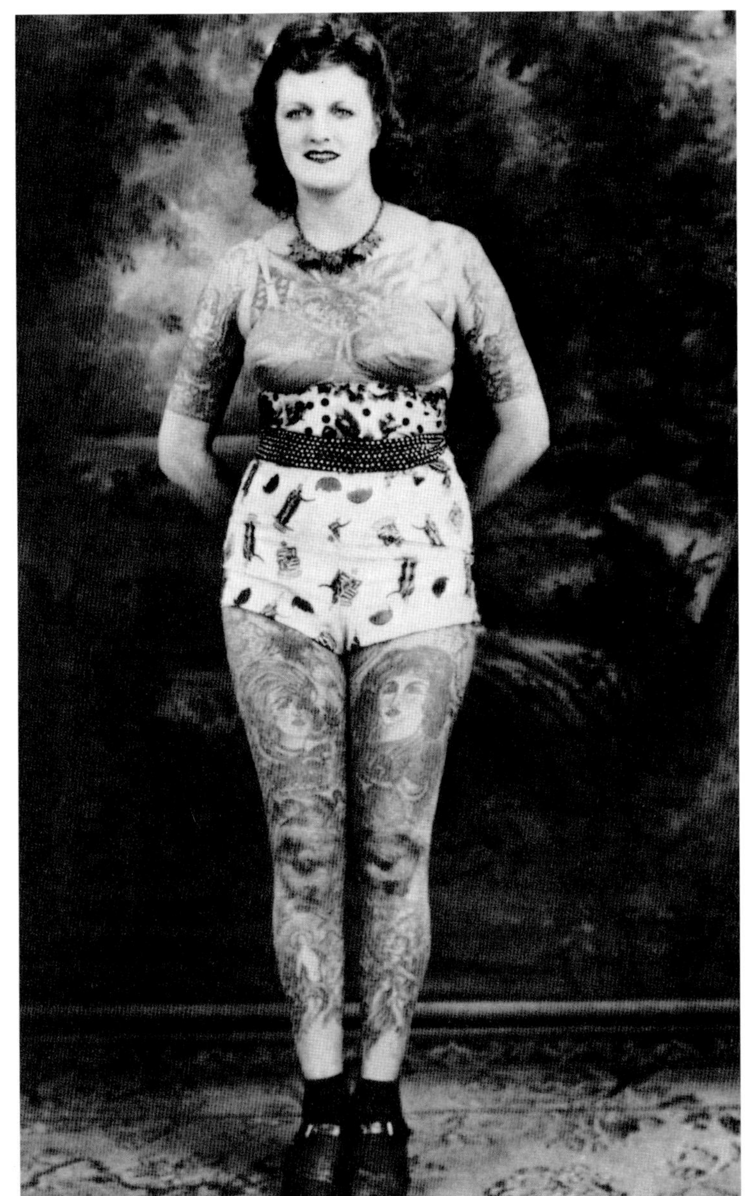

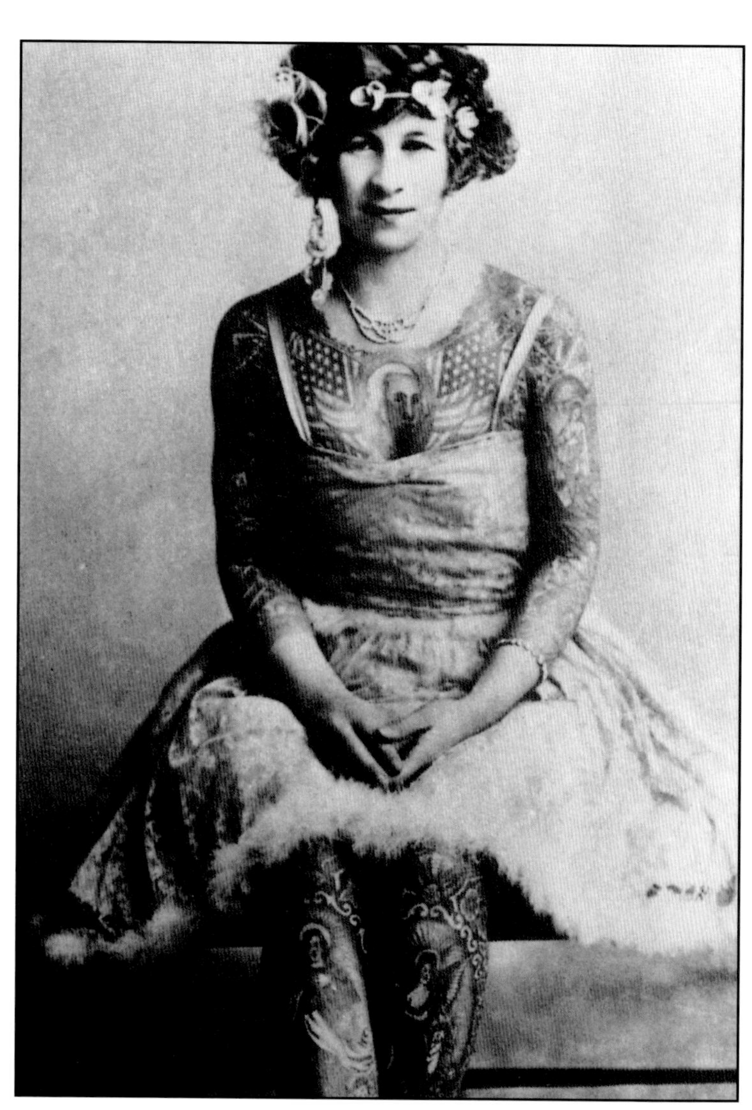

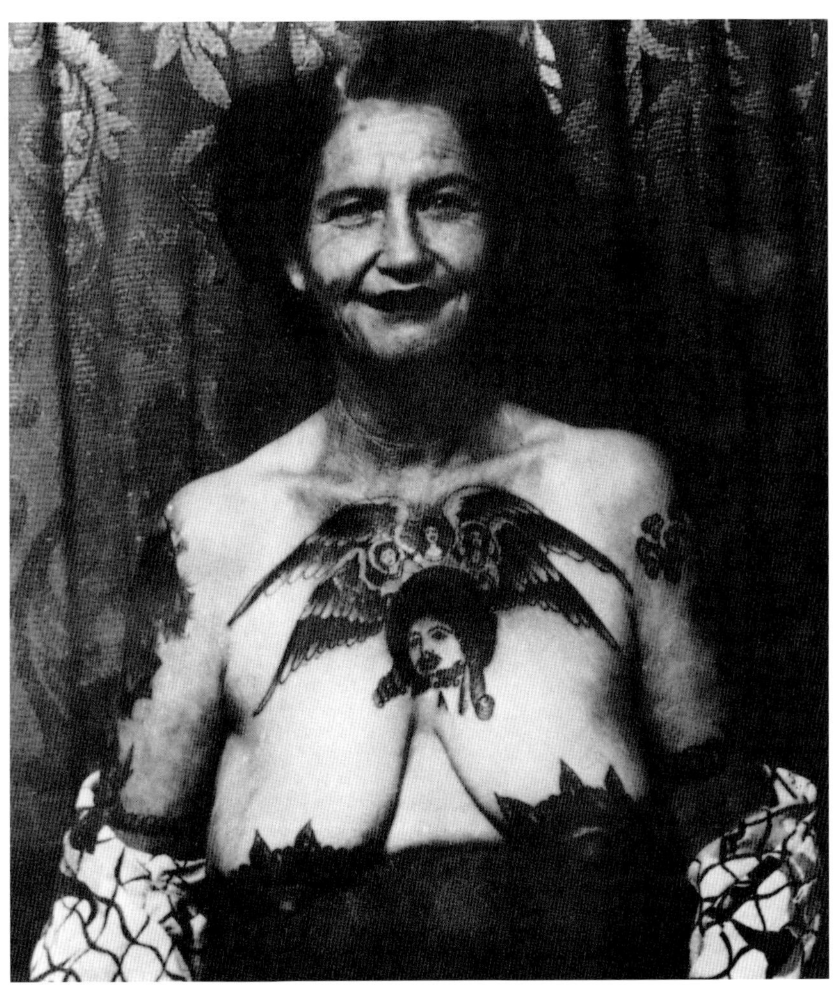

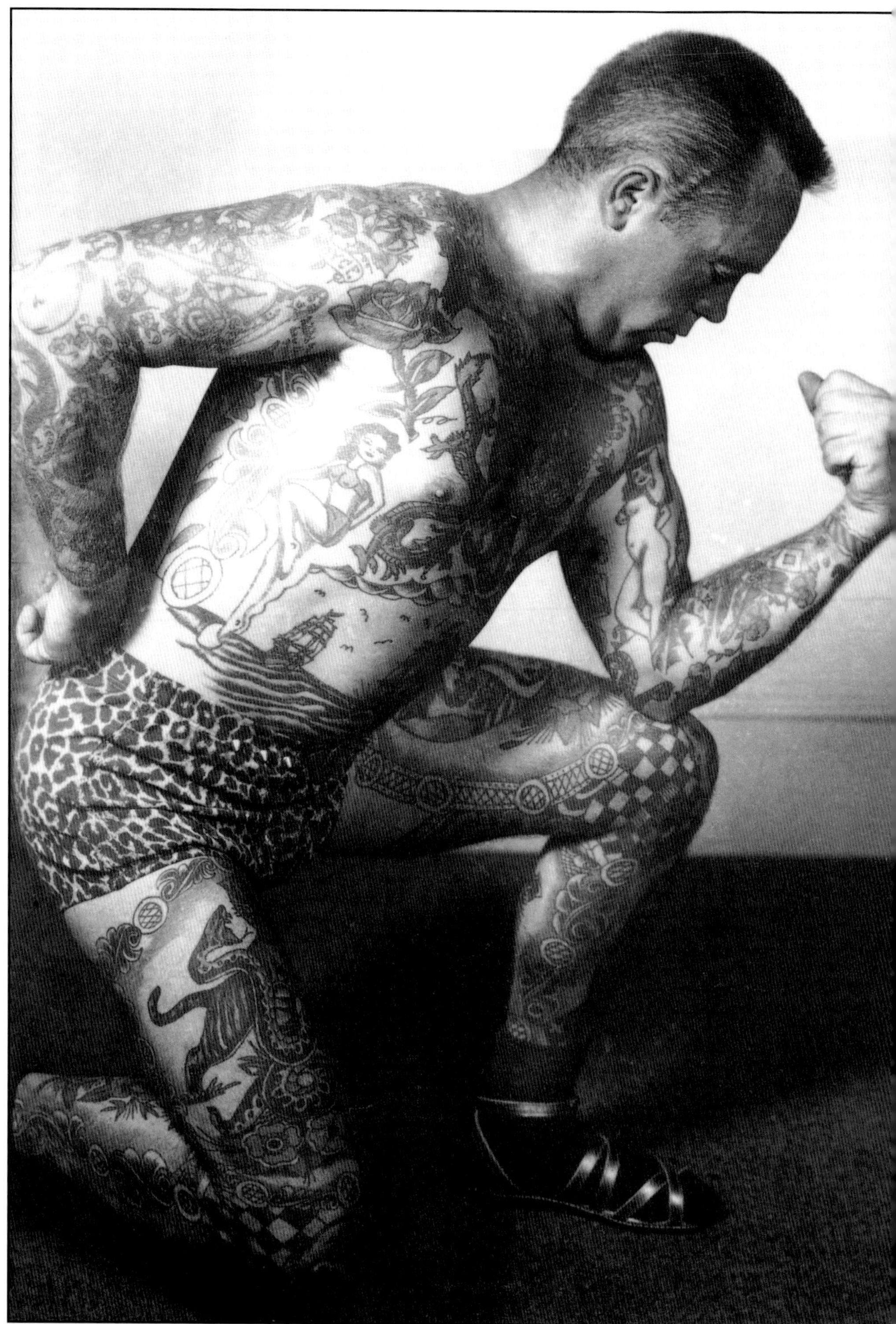

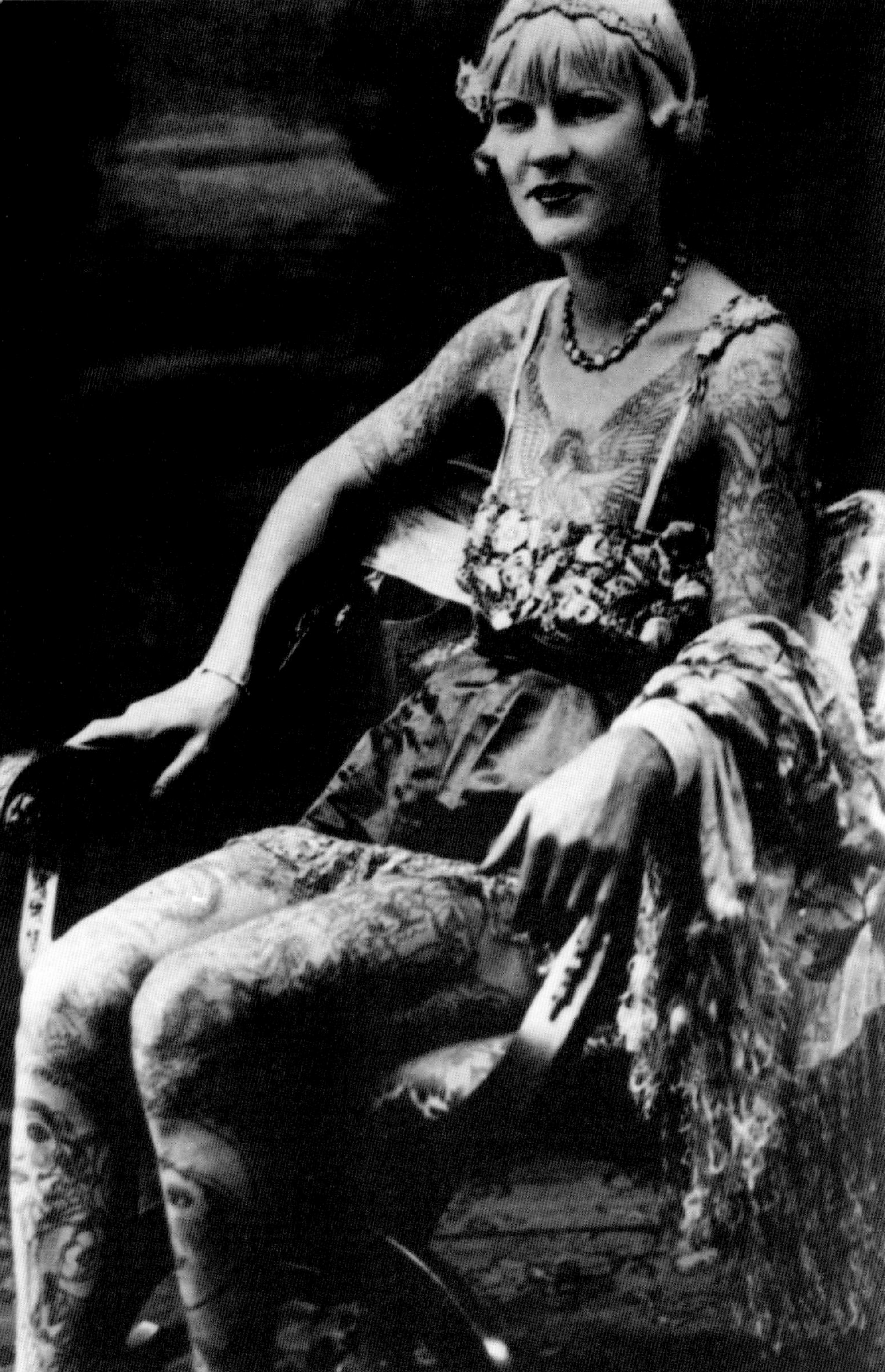

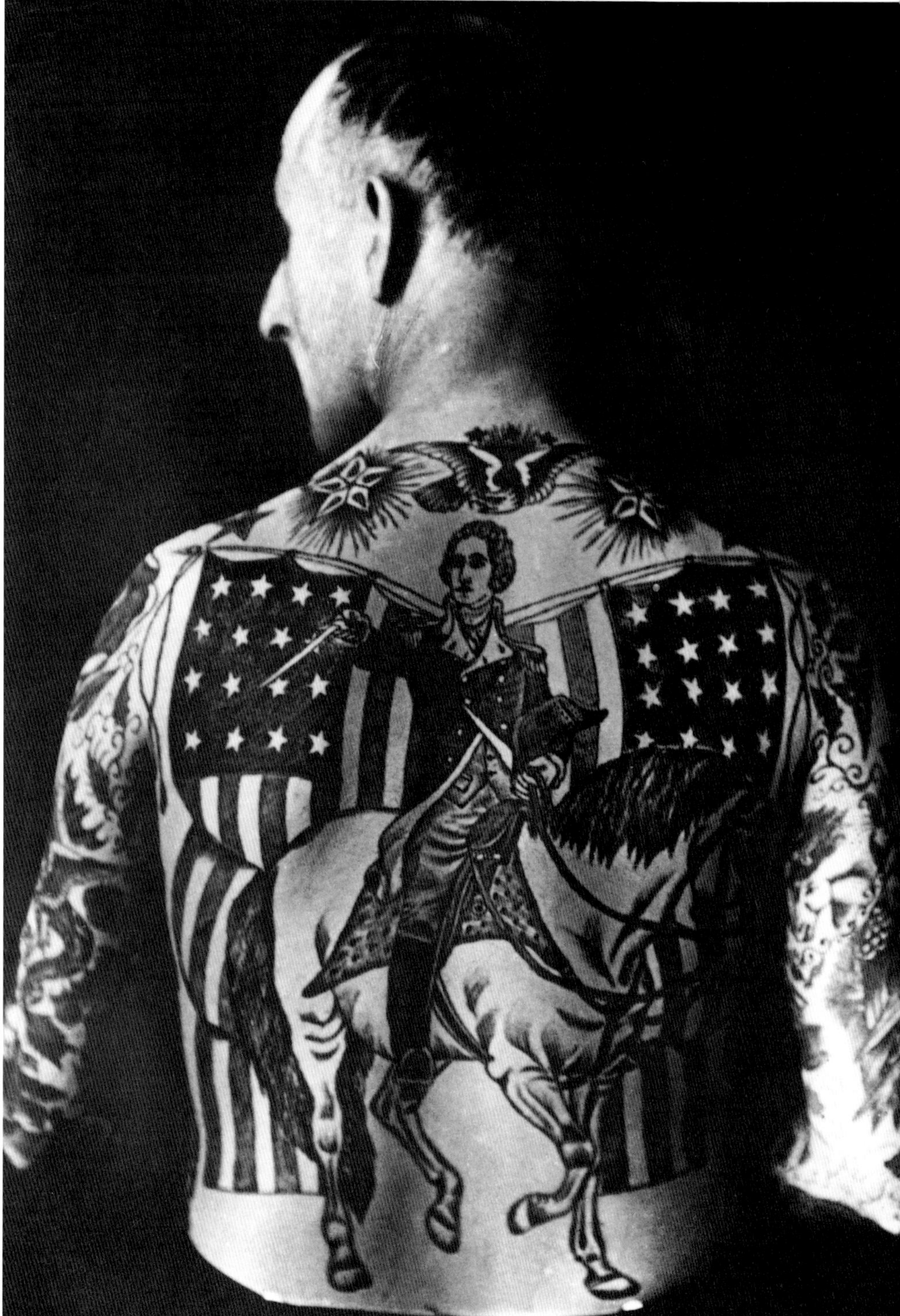

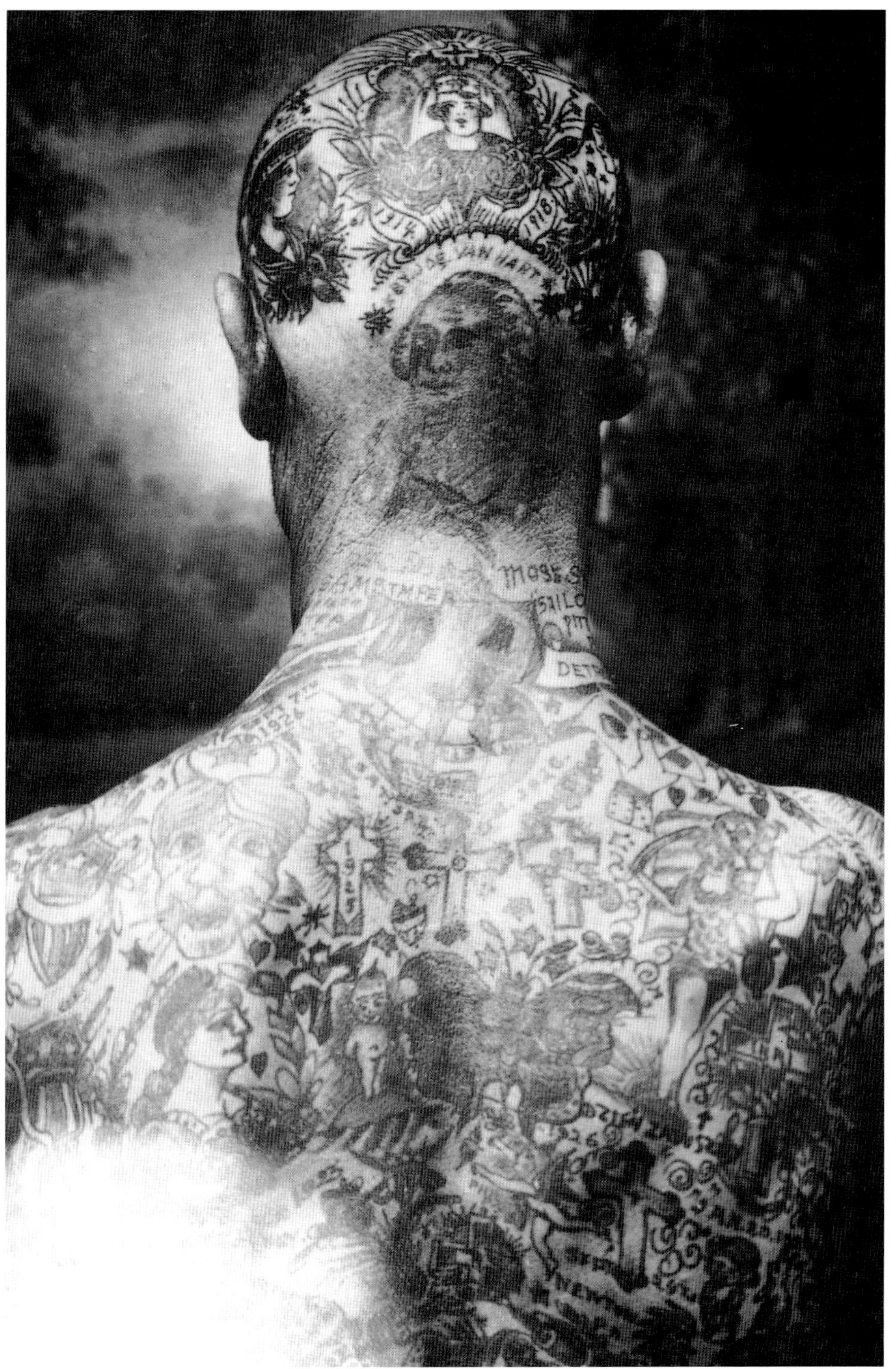

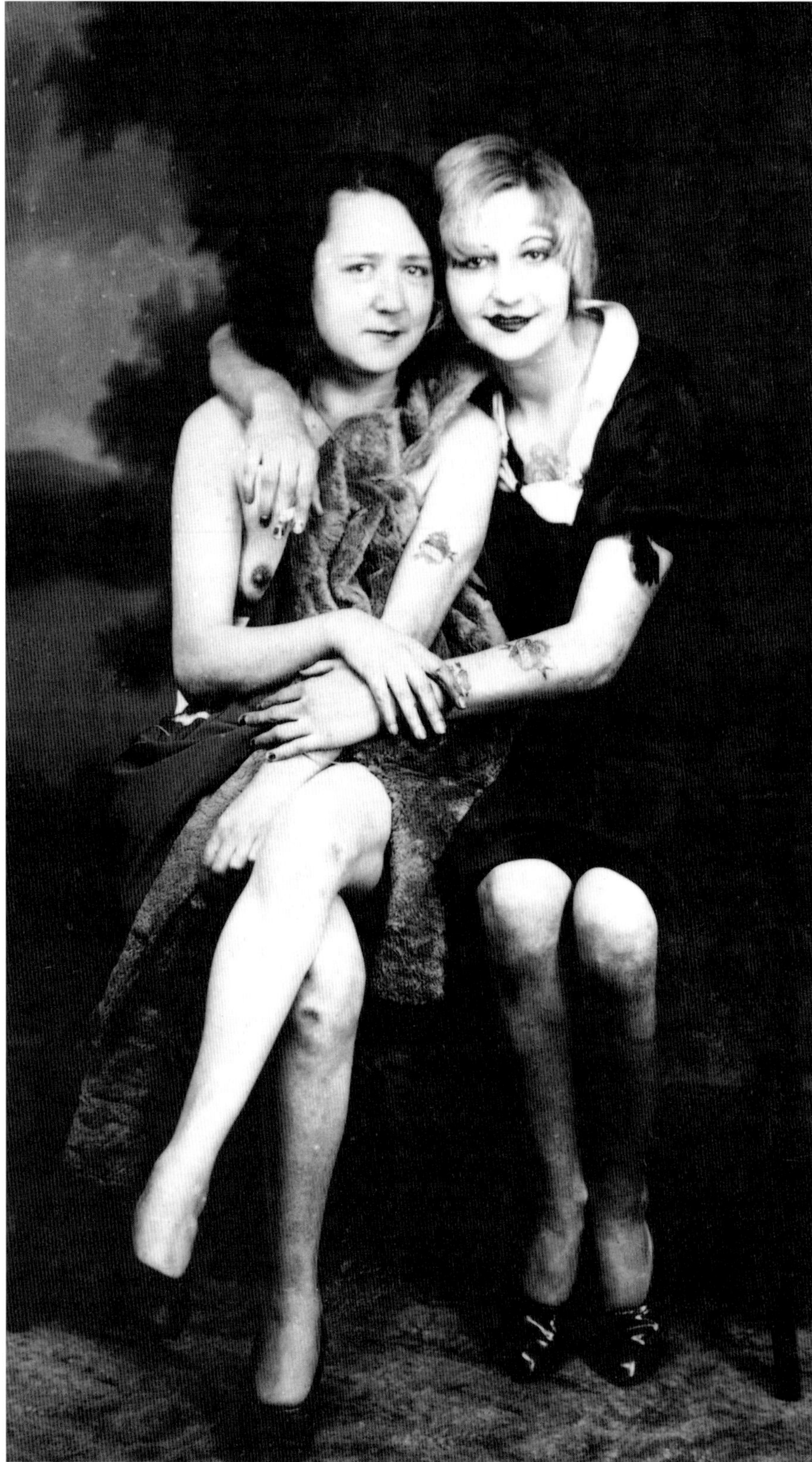

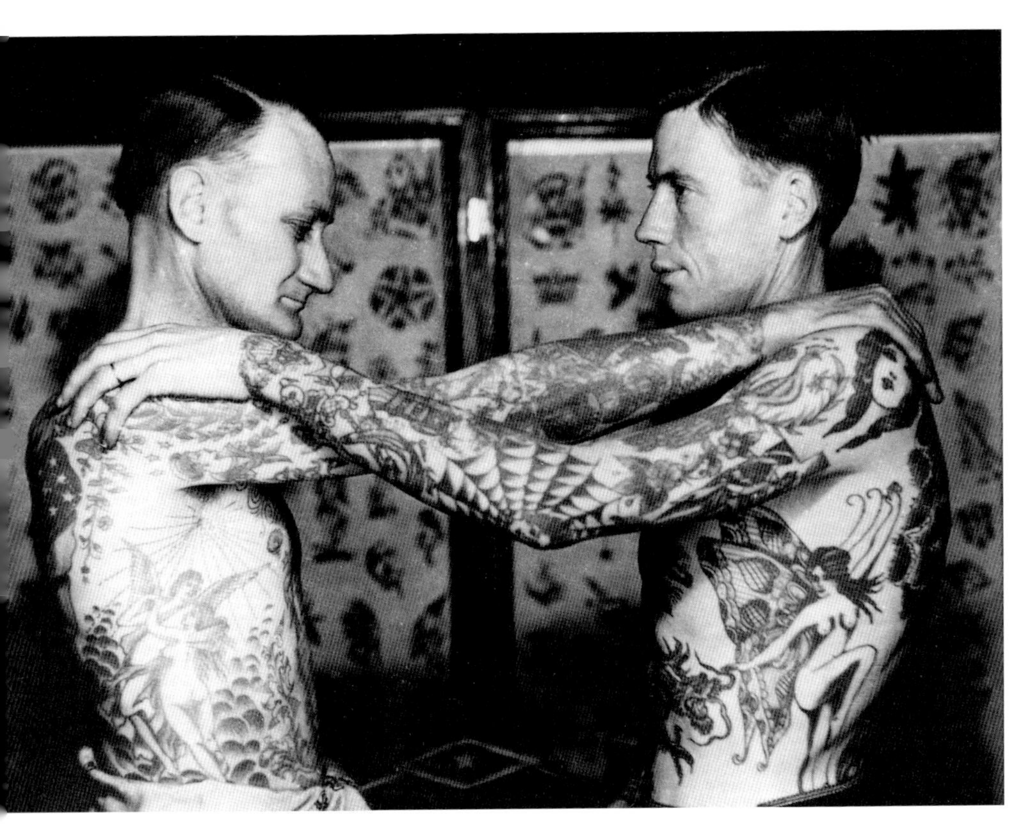

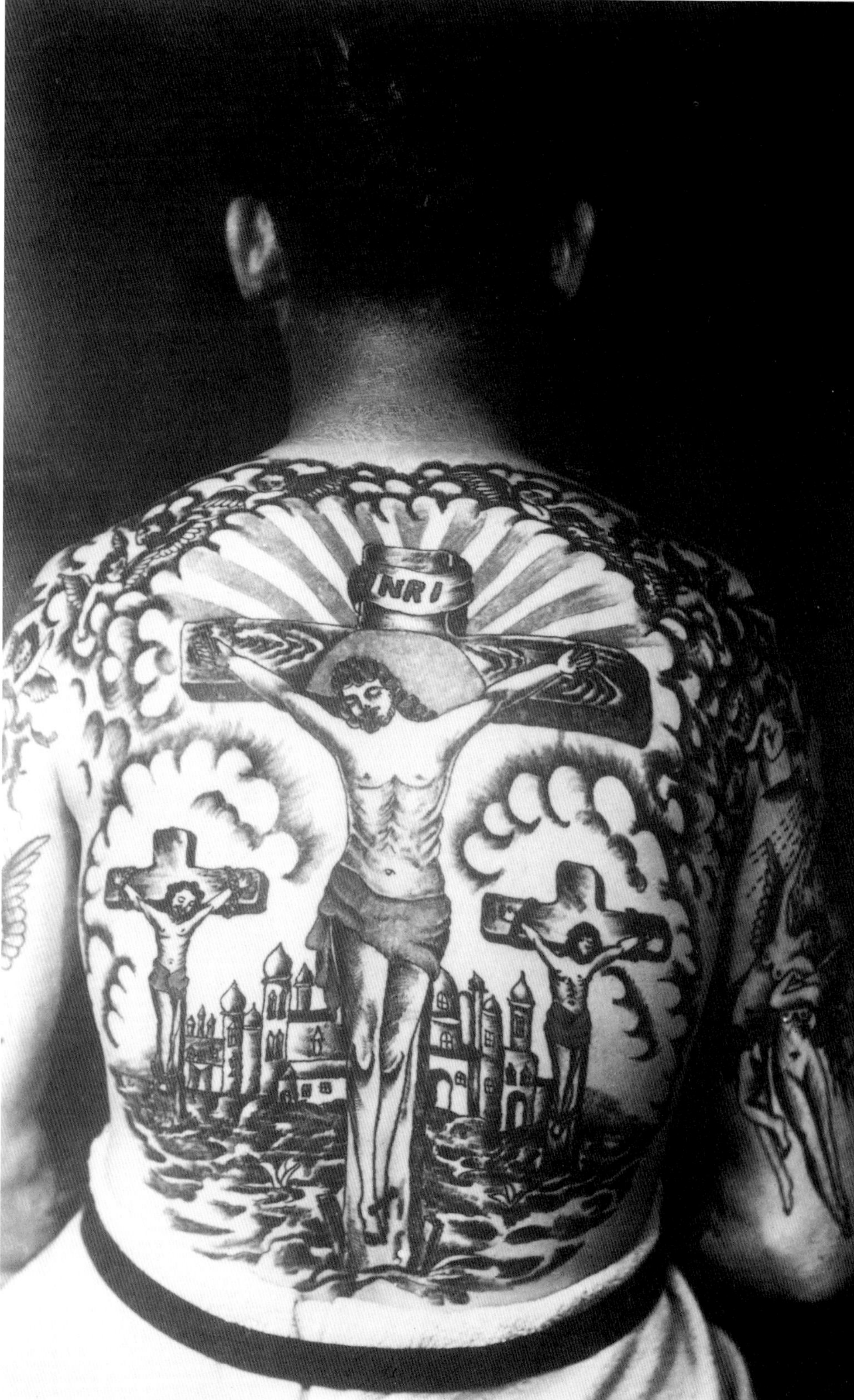

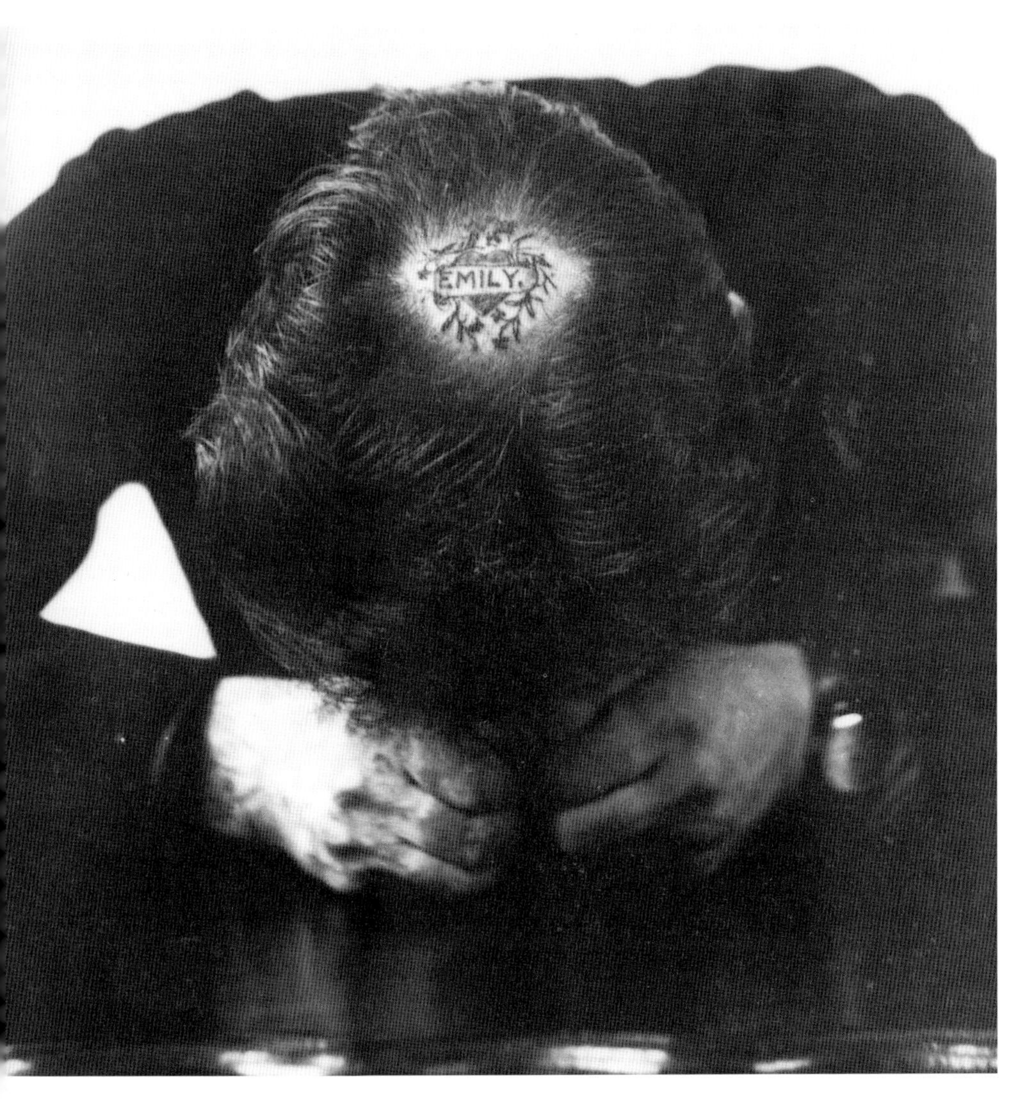

EMILY.

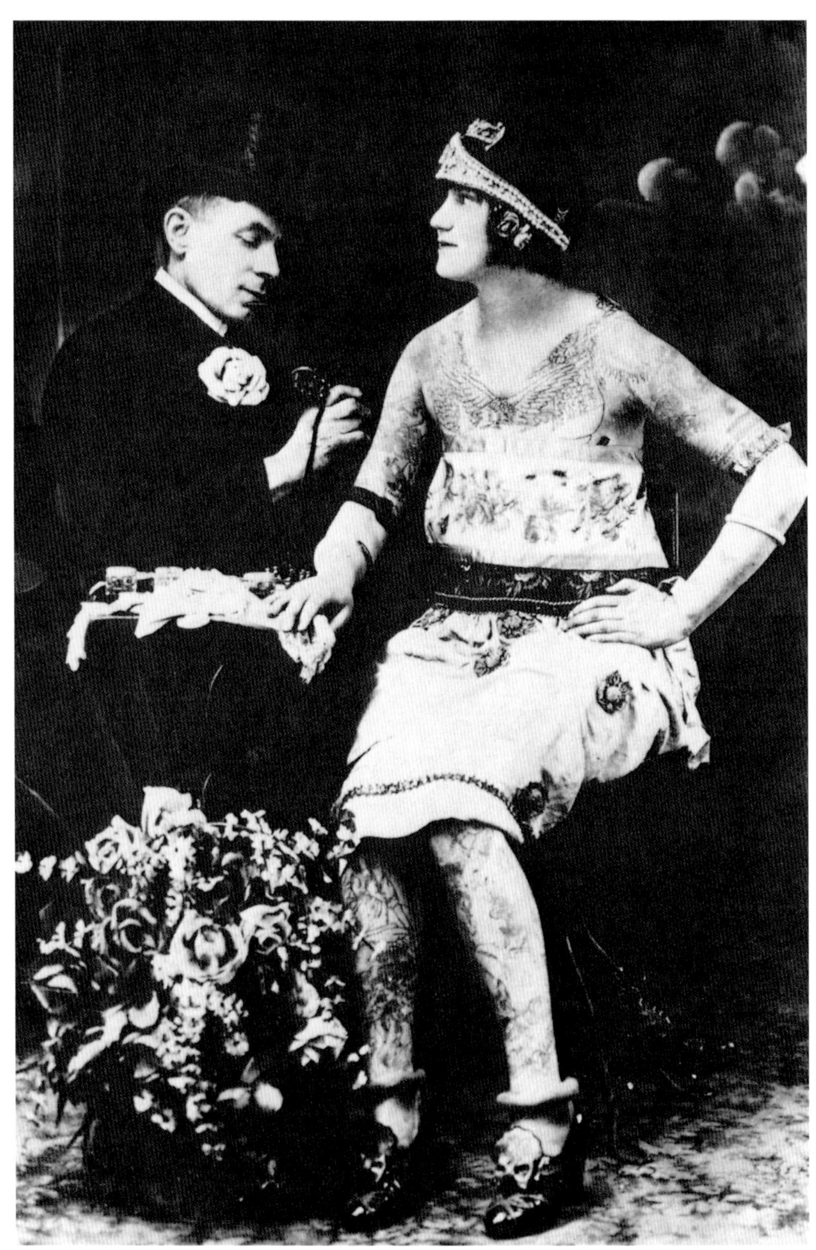

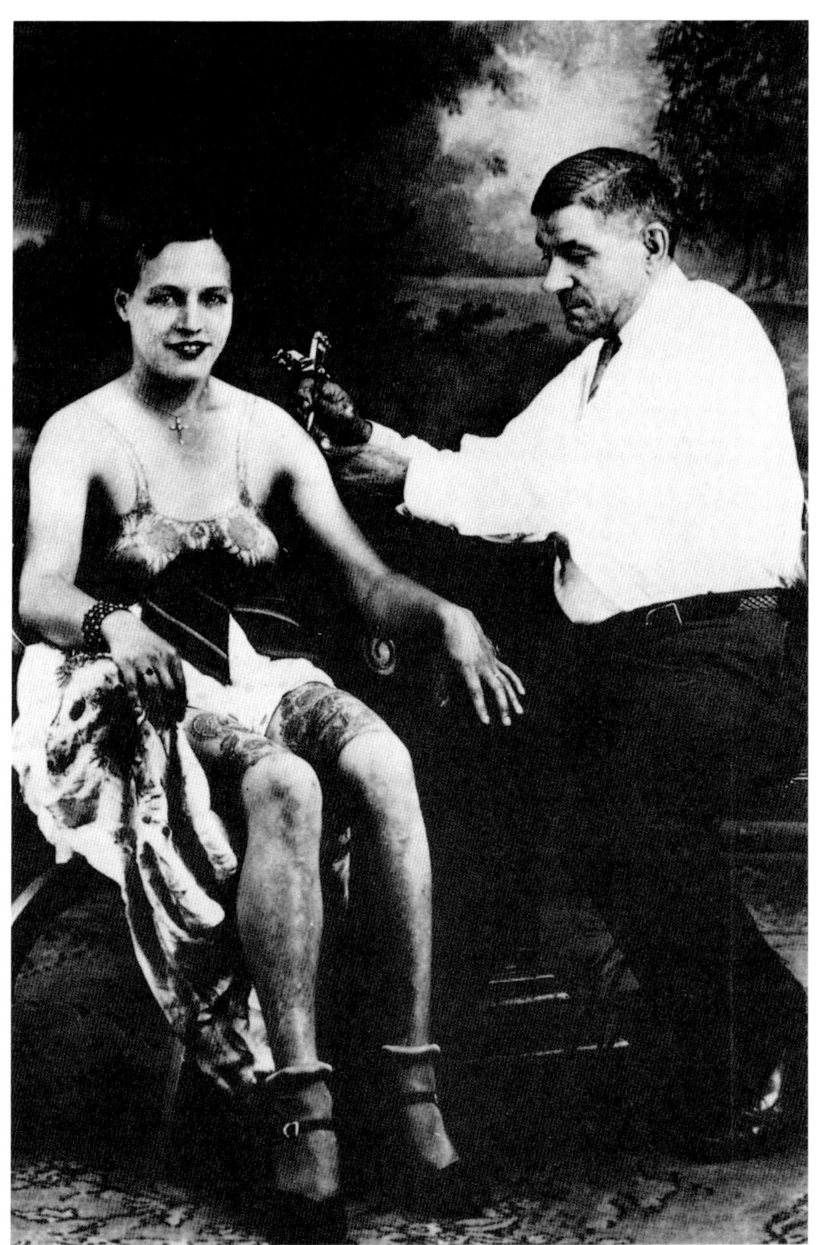

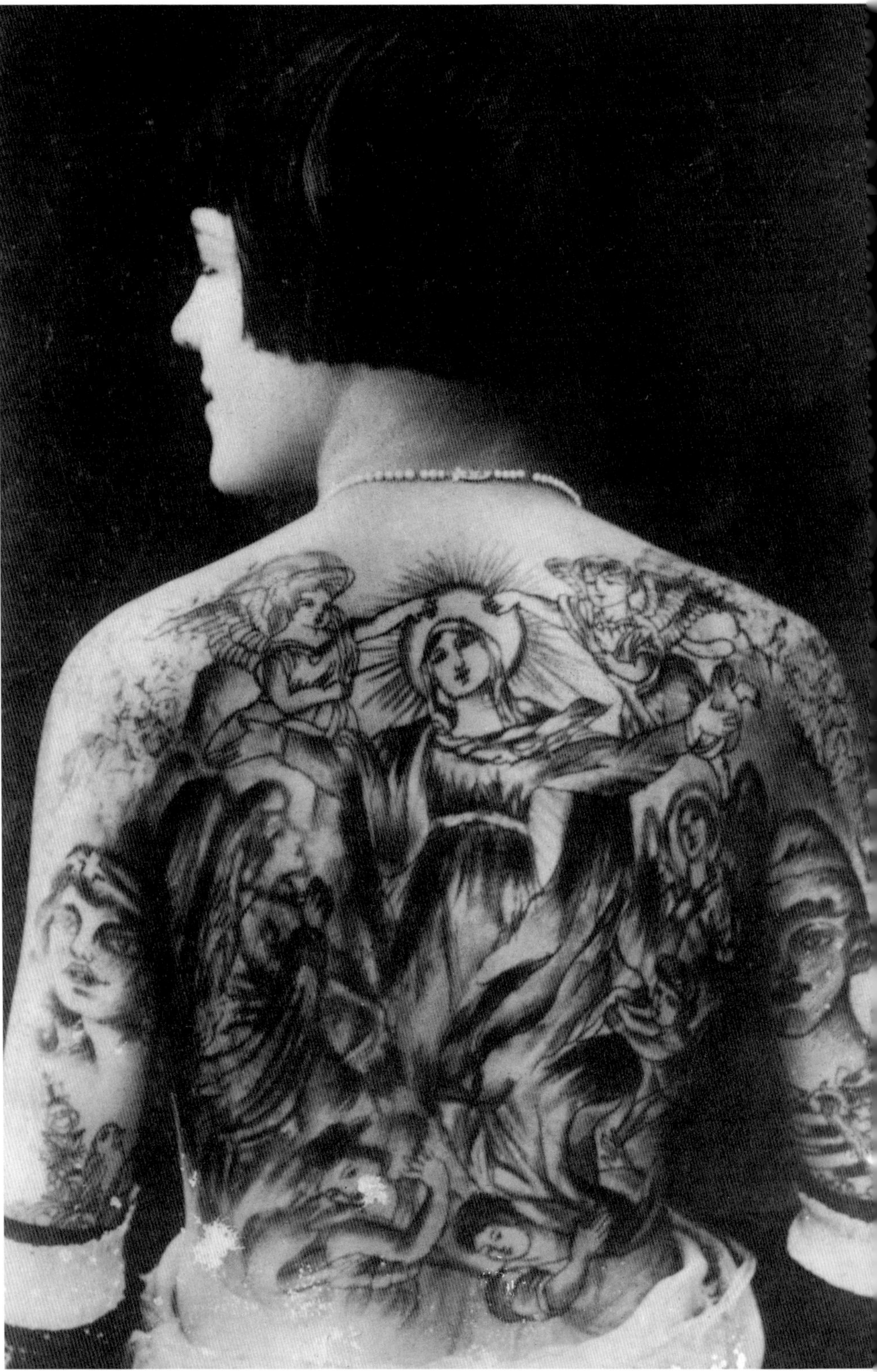

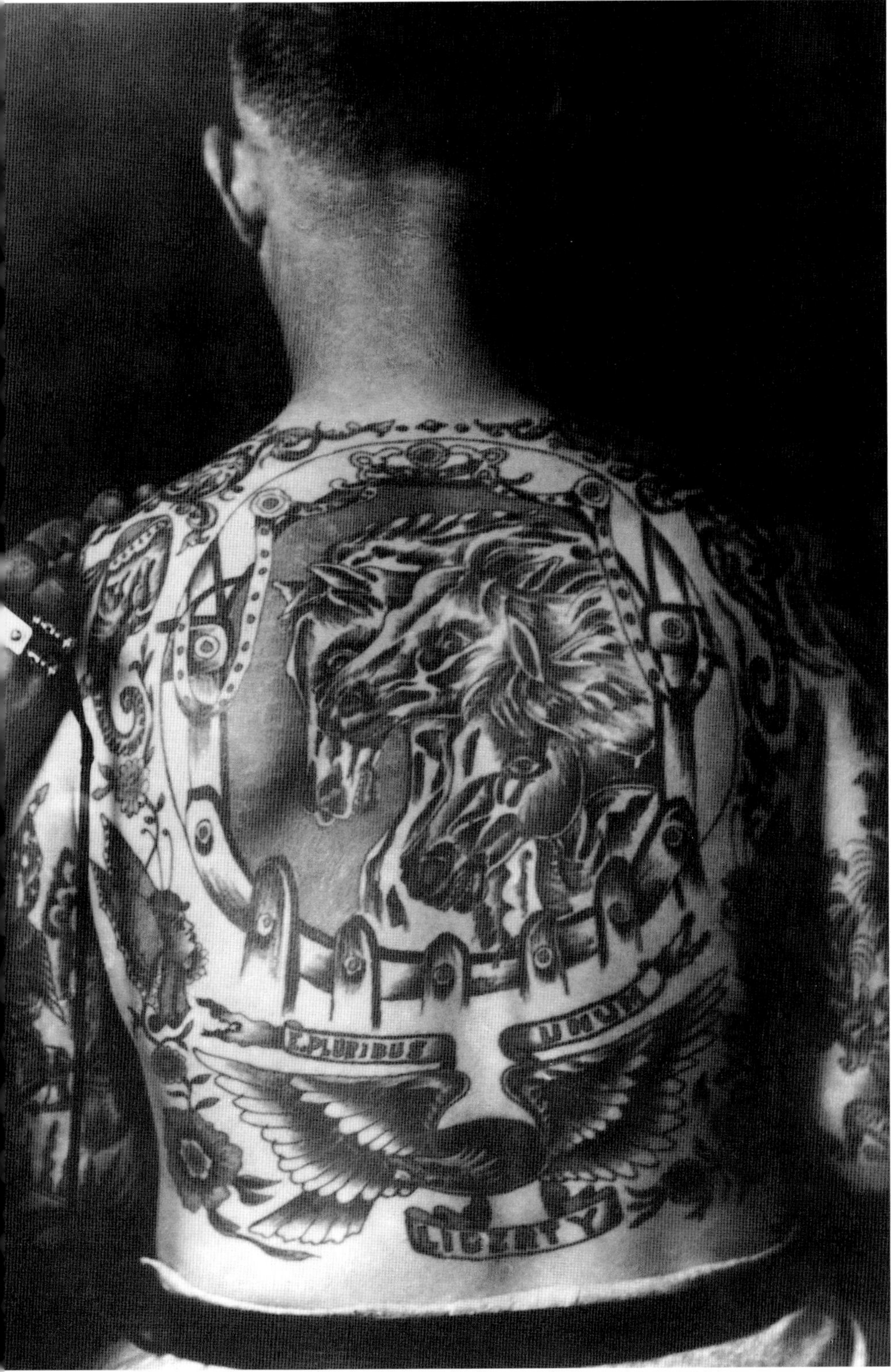

E. PLURIBUS
LIBERTY

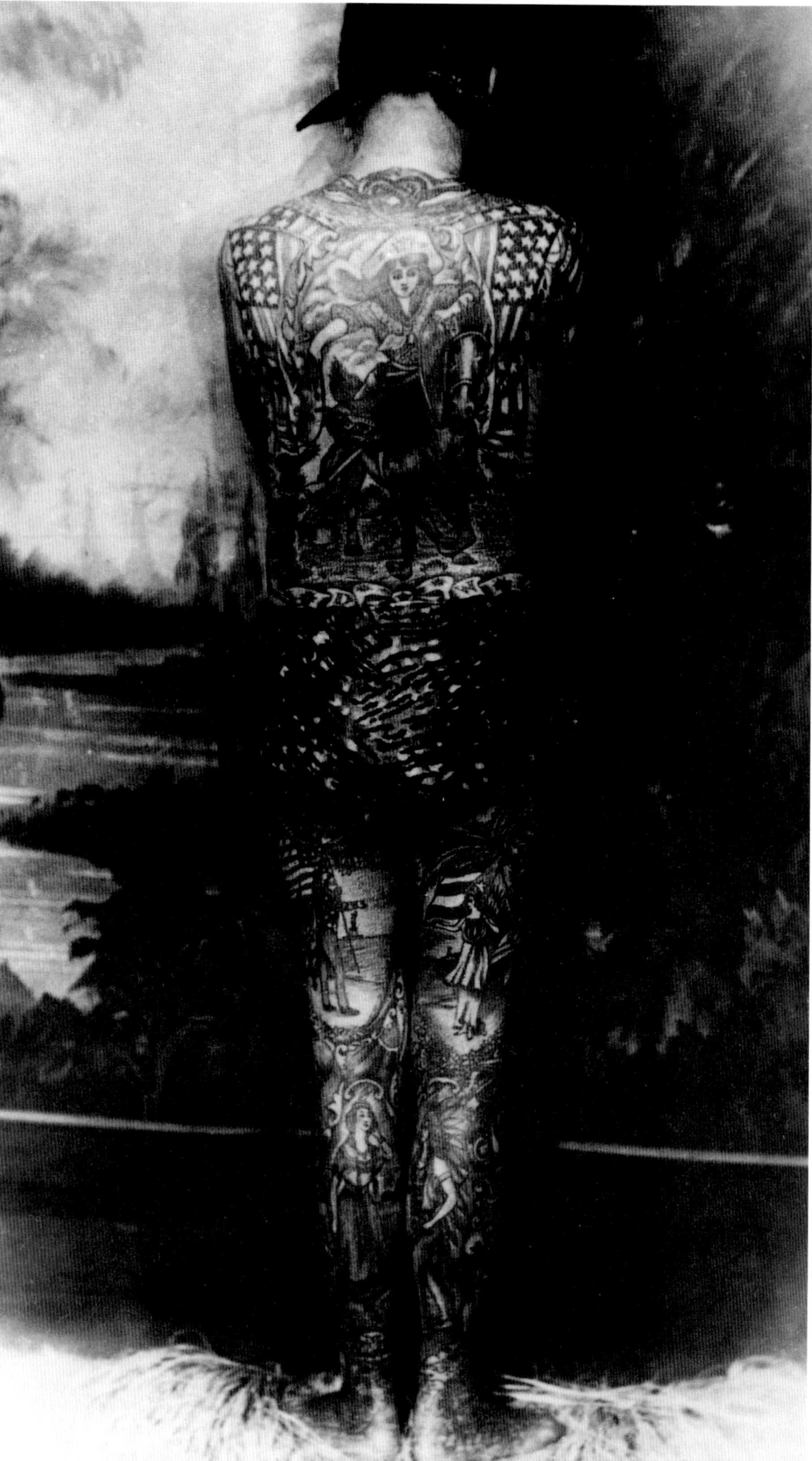

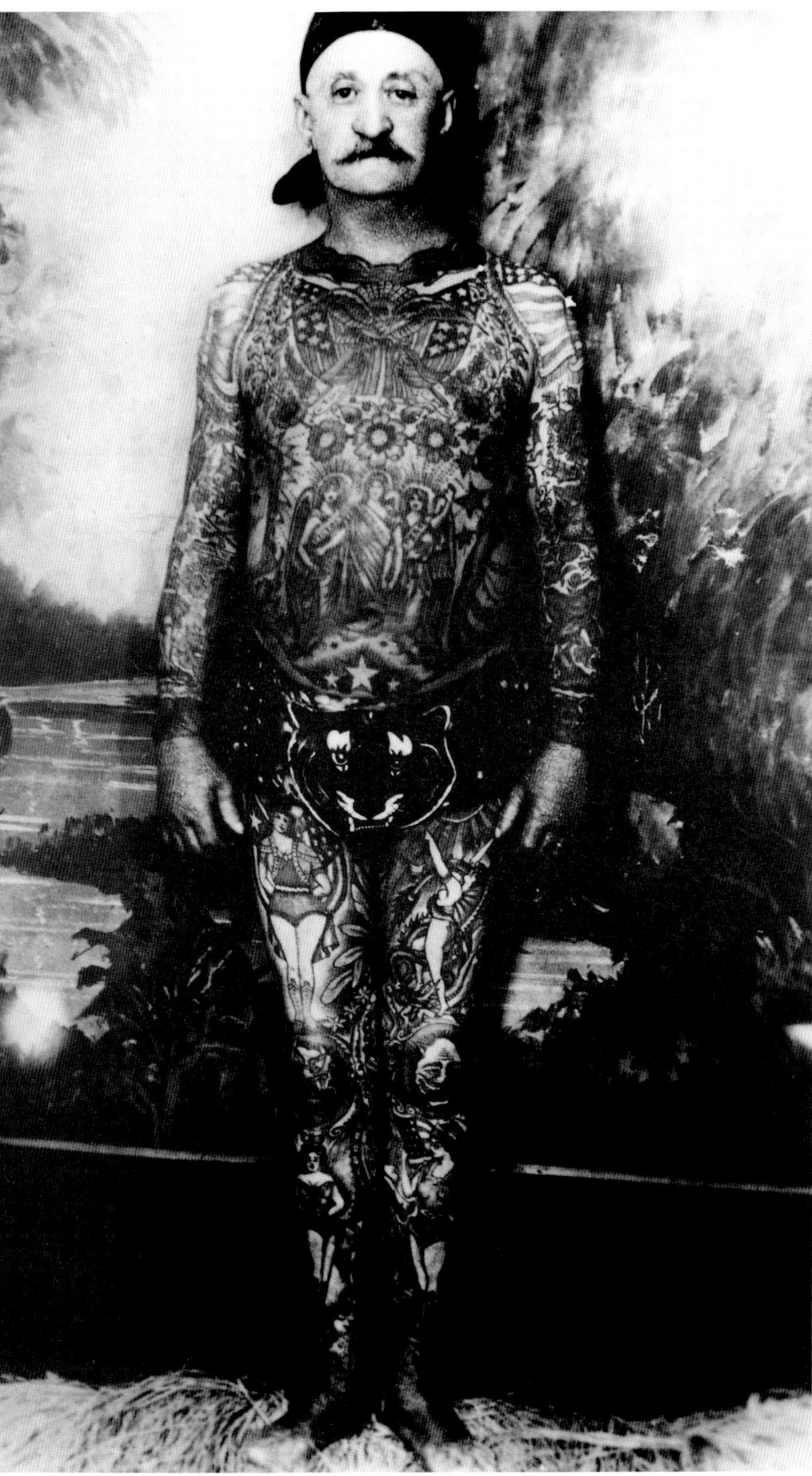

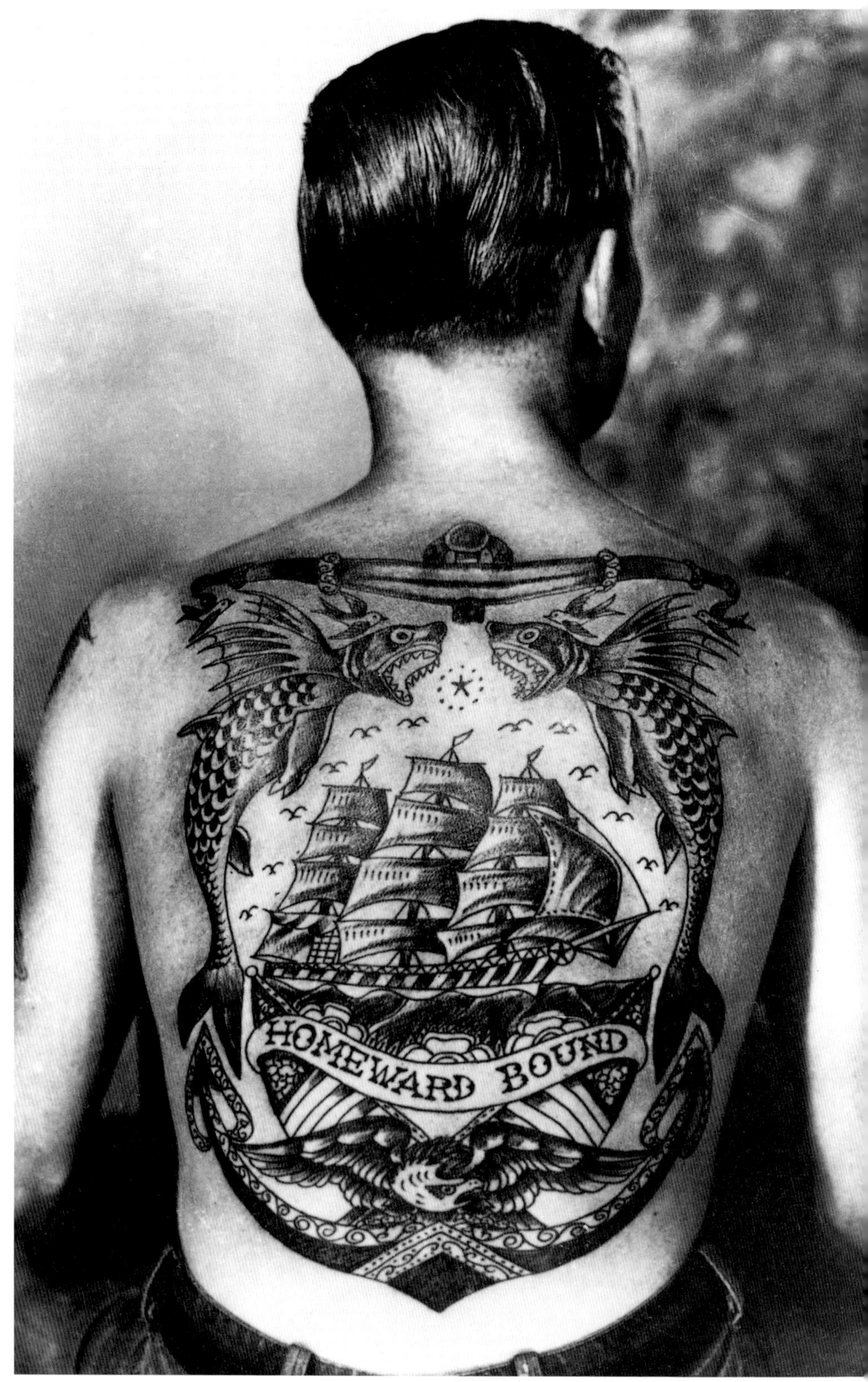

HOMEWARD BOUND

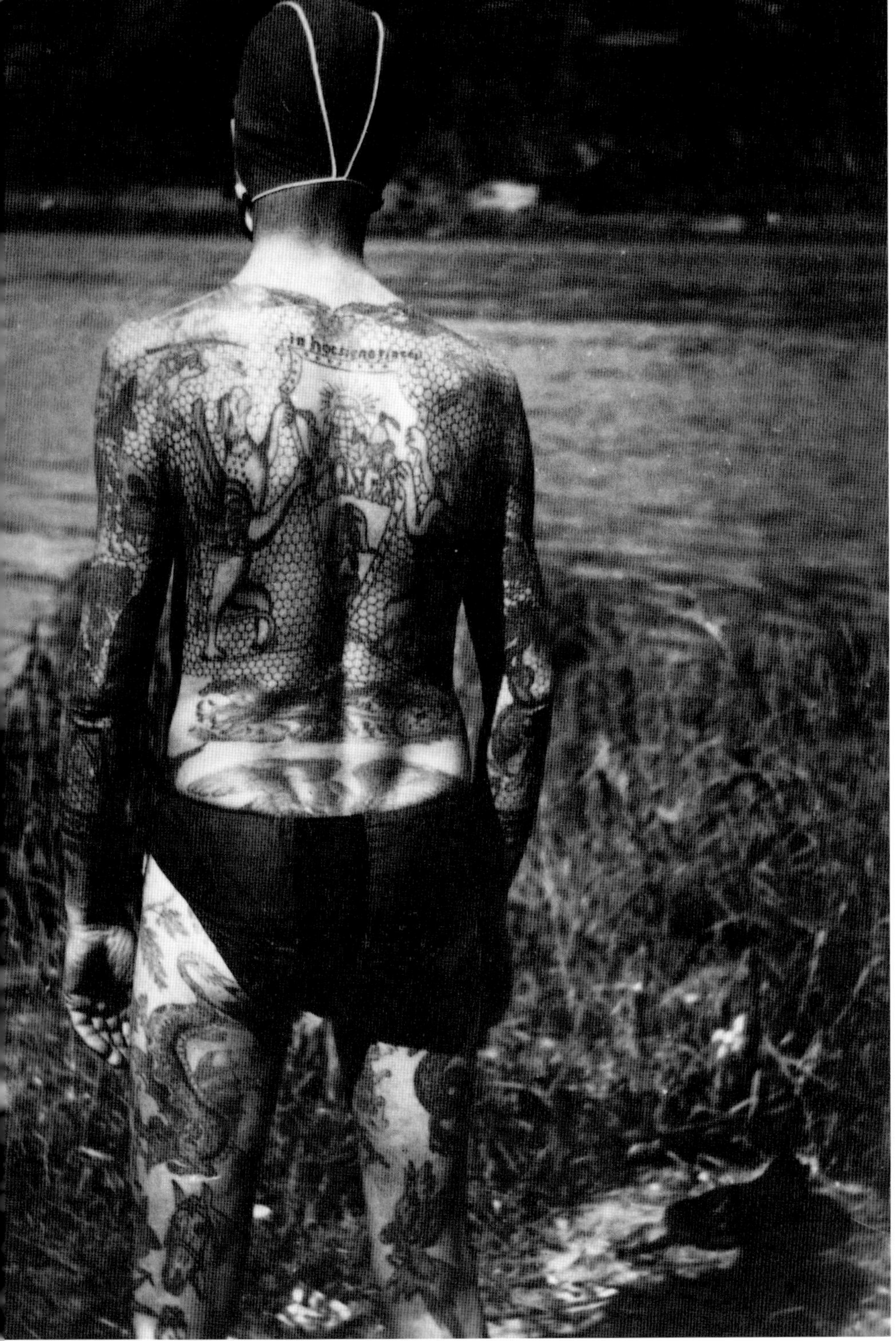

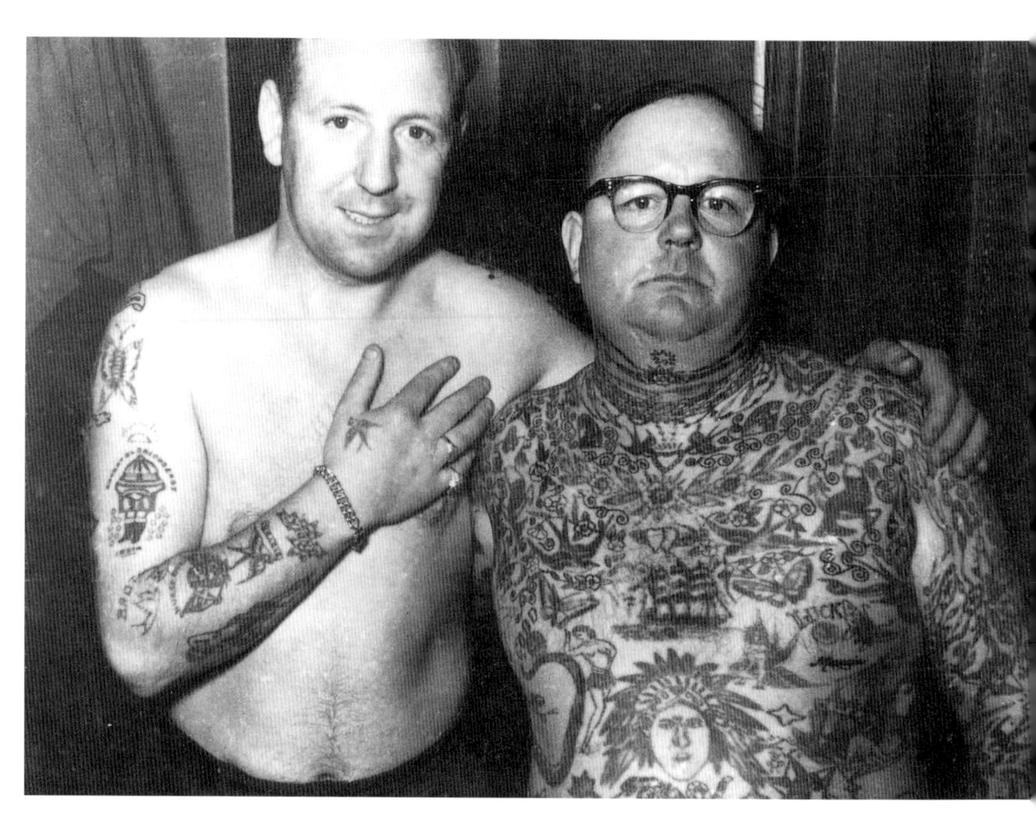

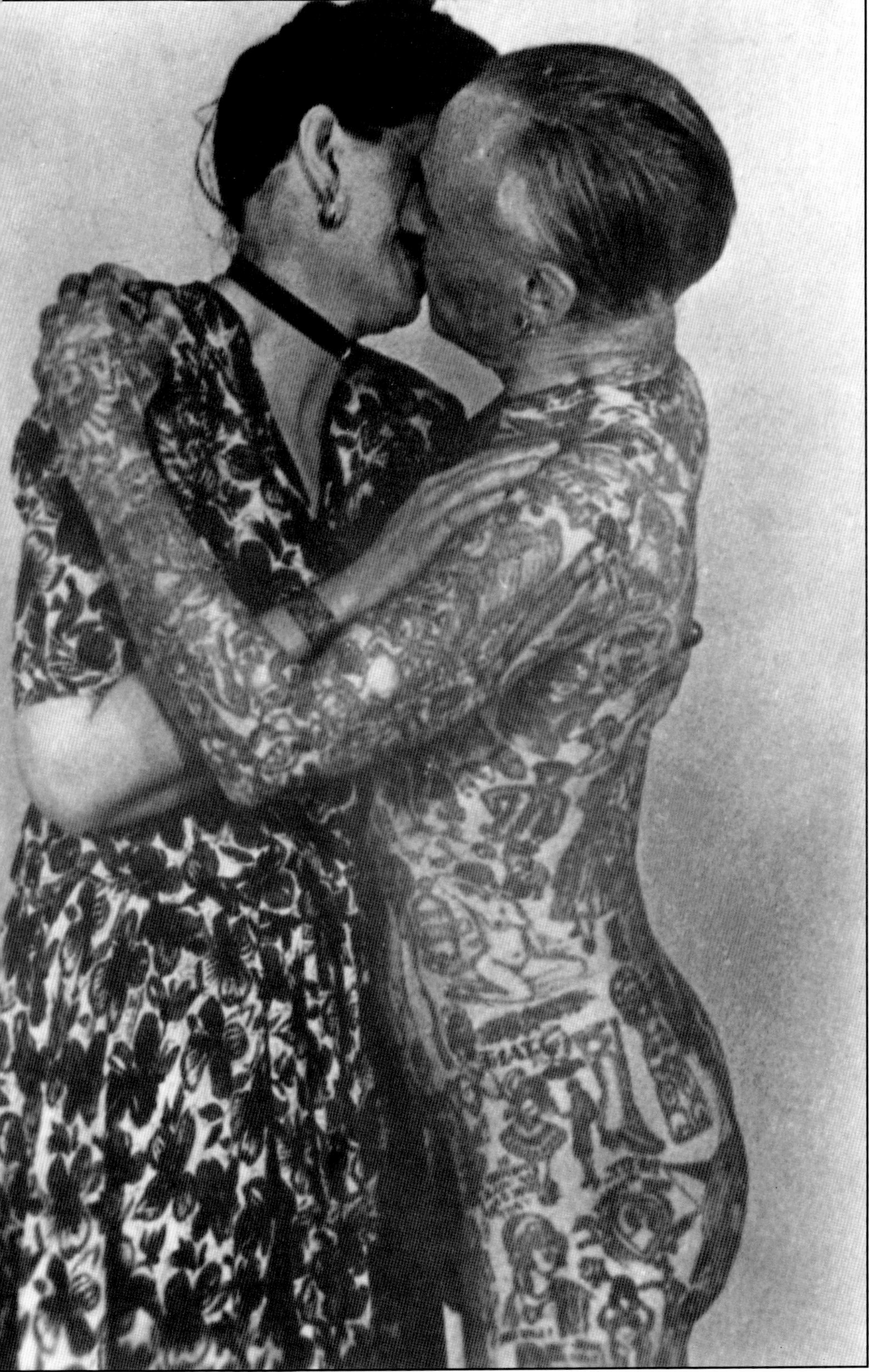

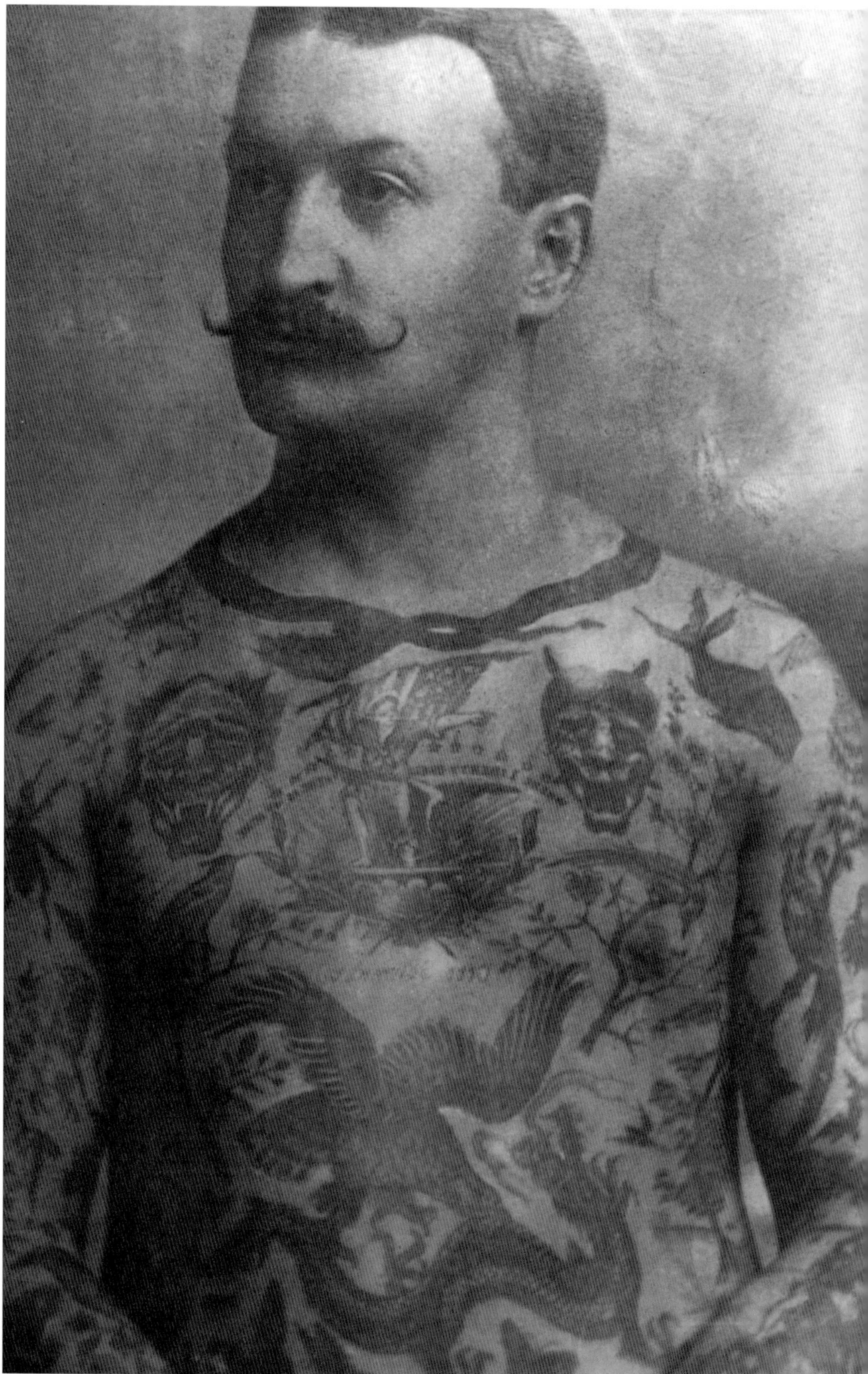

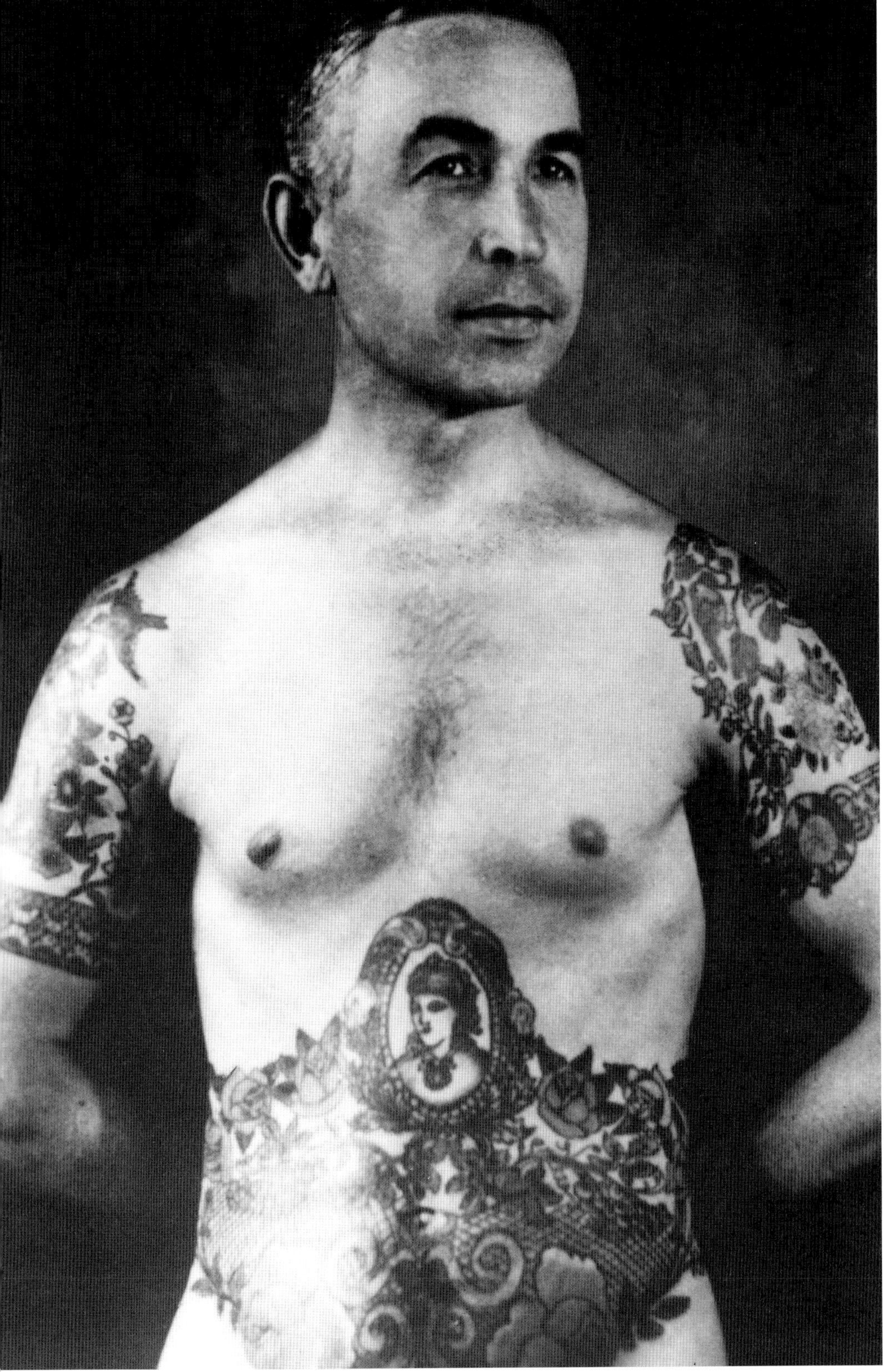

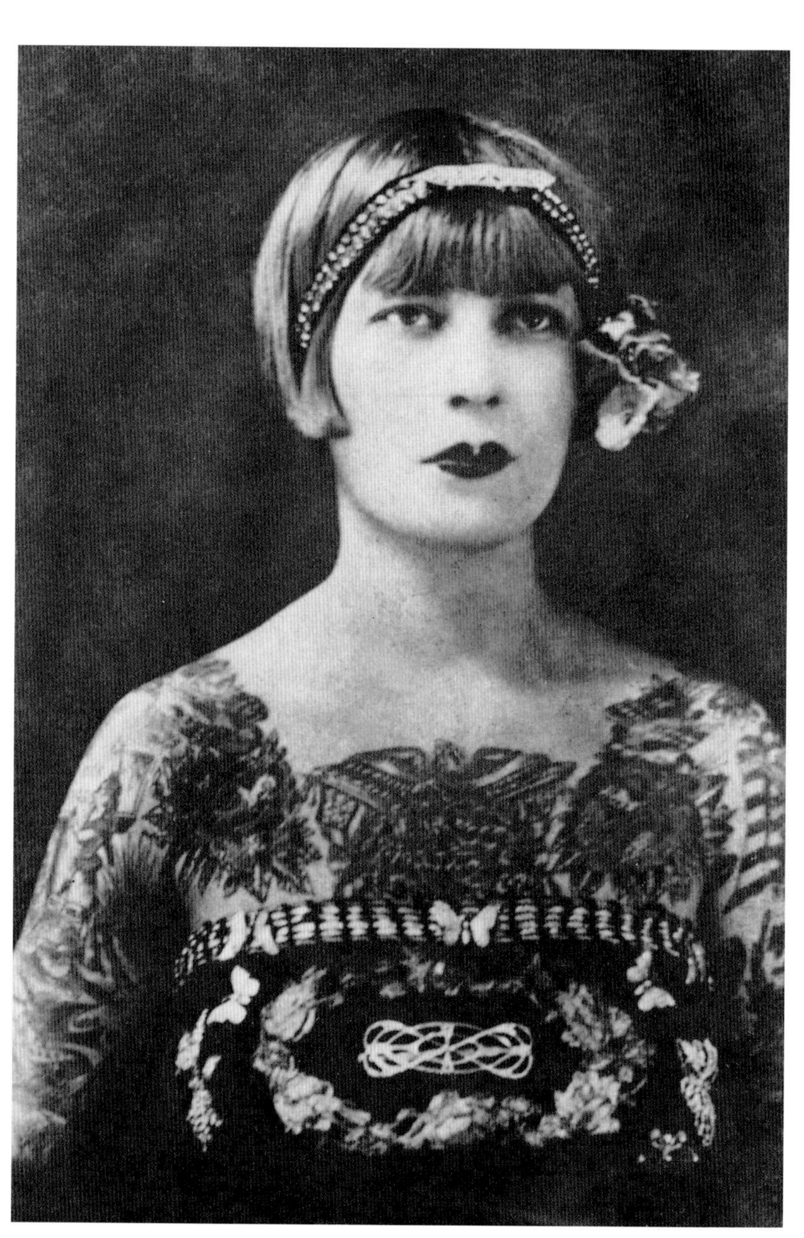

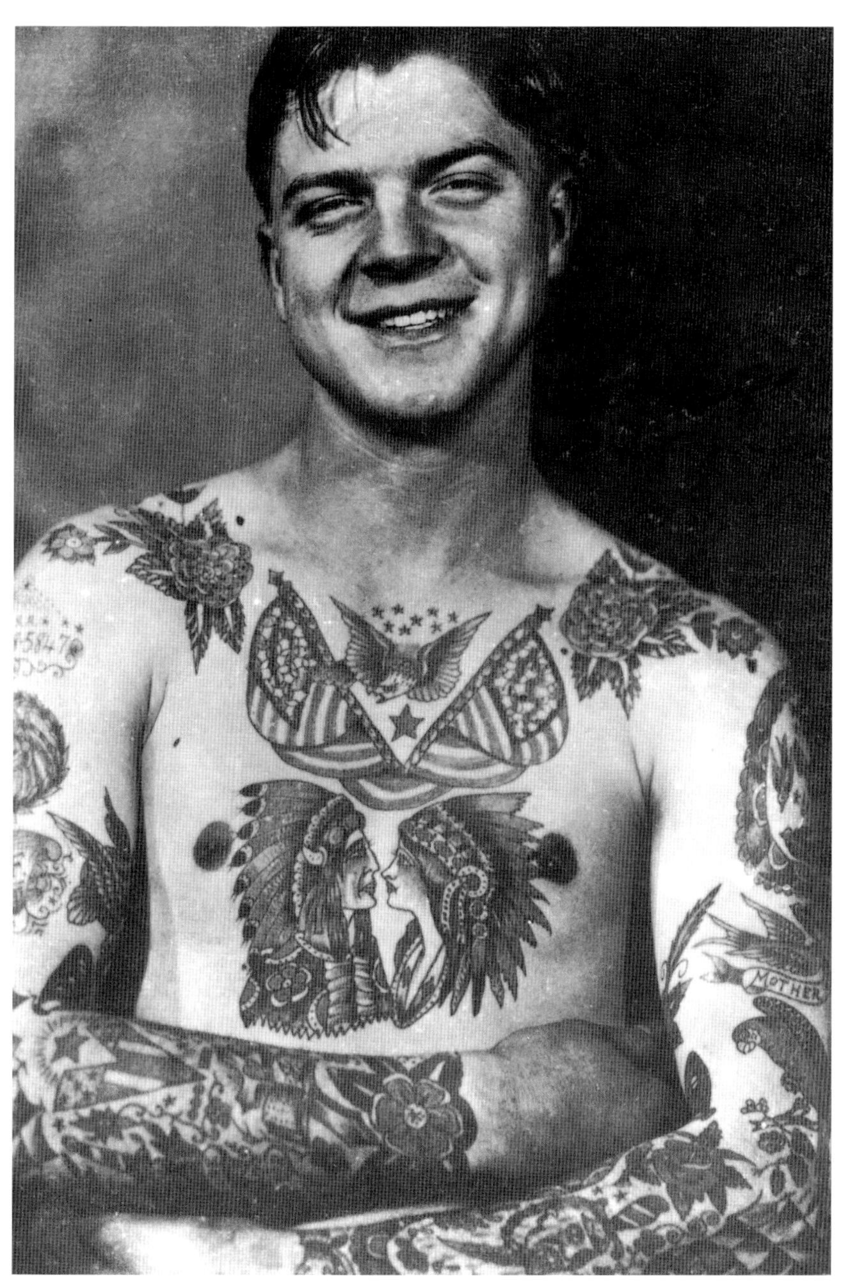
MOTHER

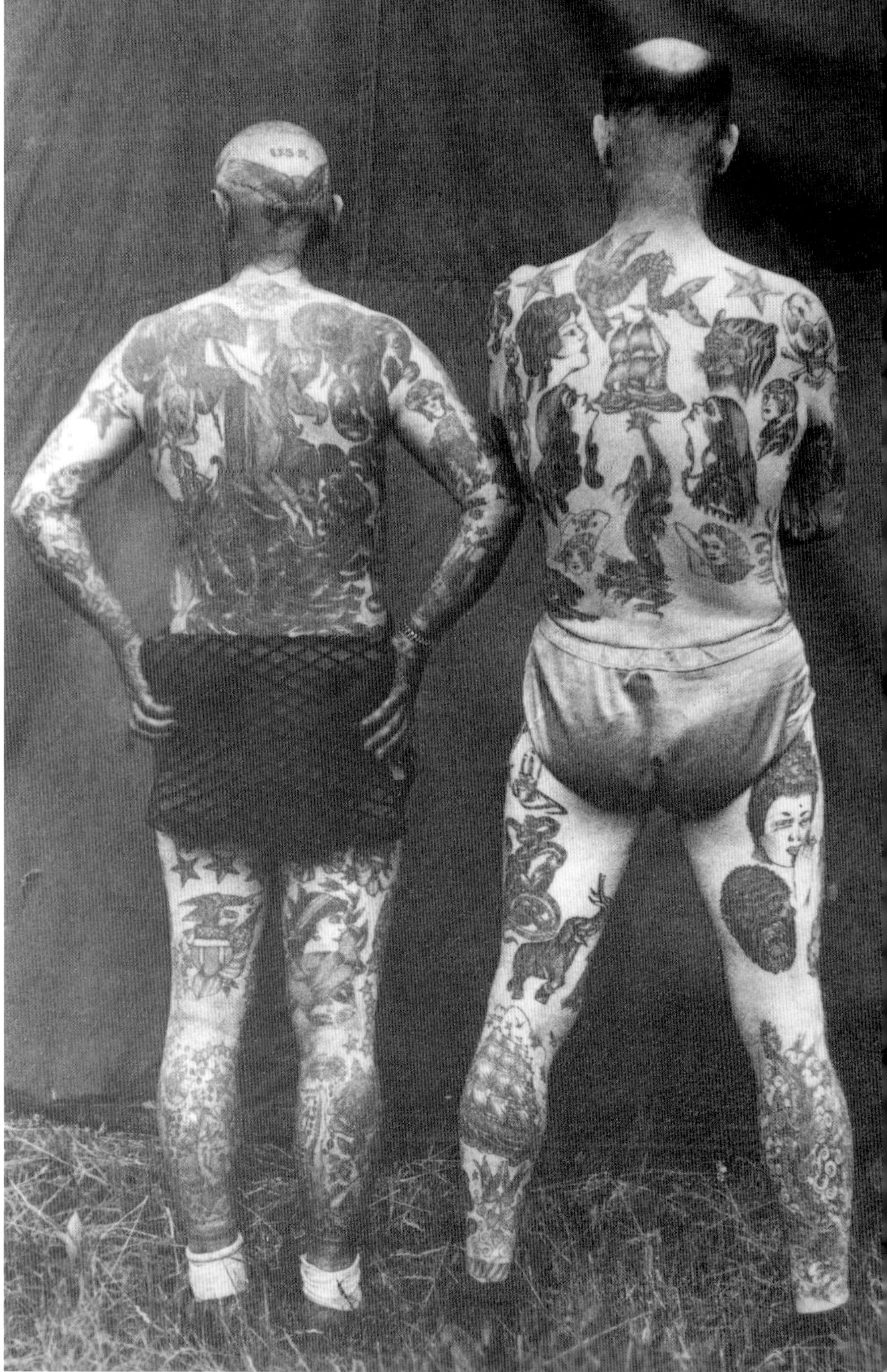

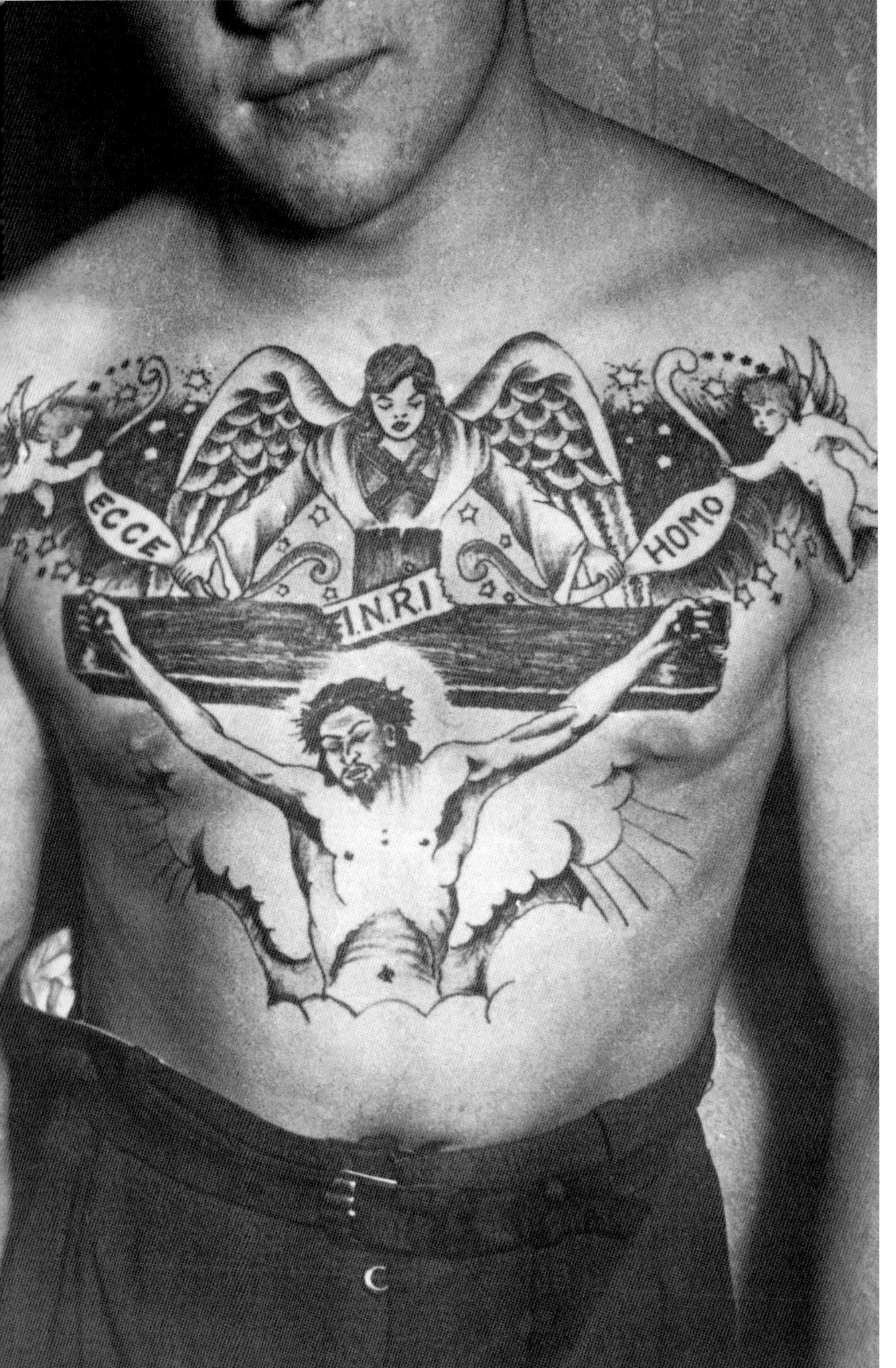
ECCE
HOMO
I.N.R.I

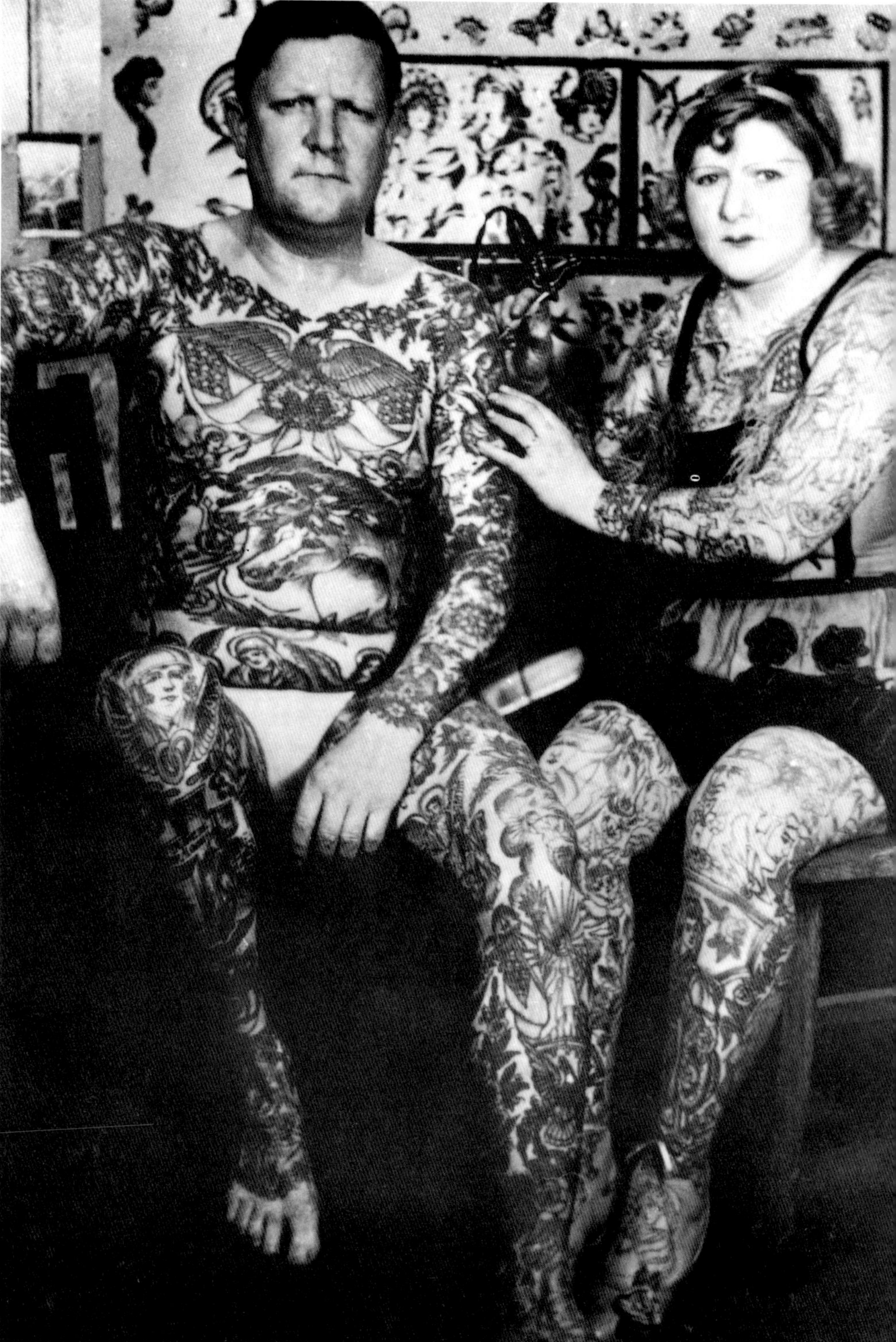

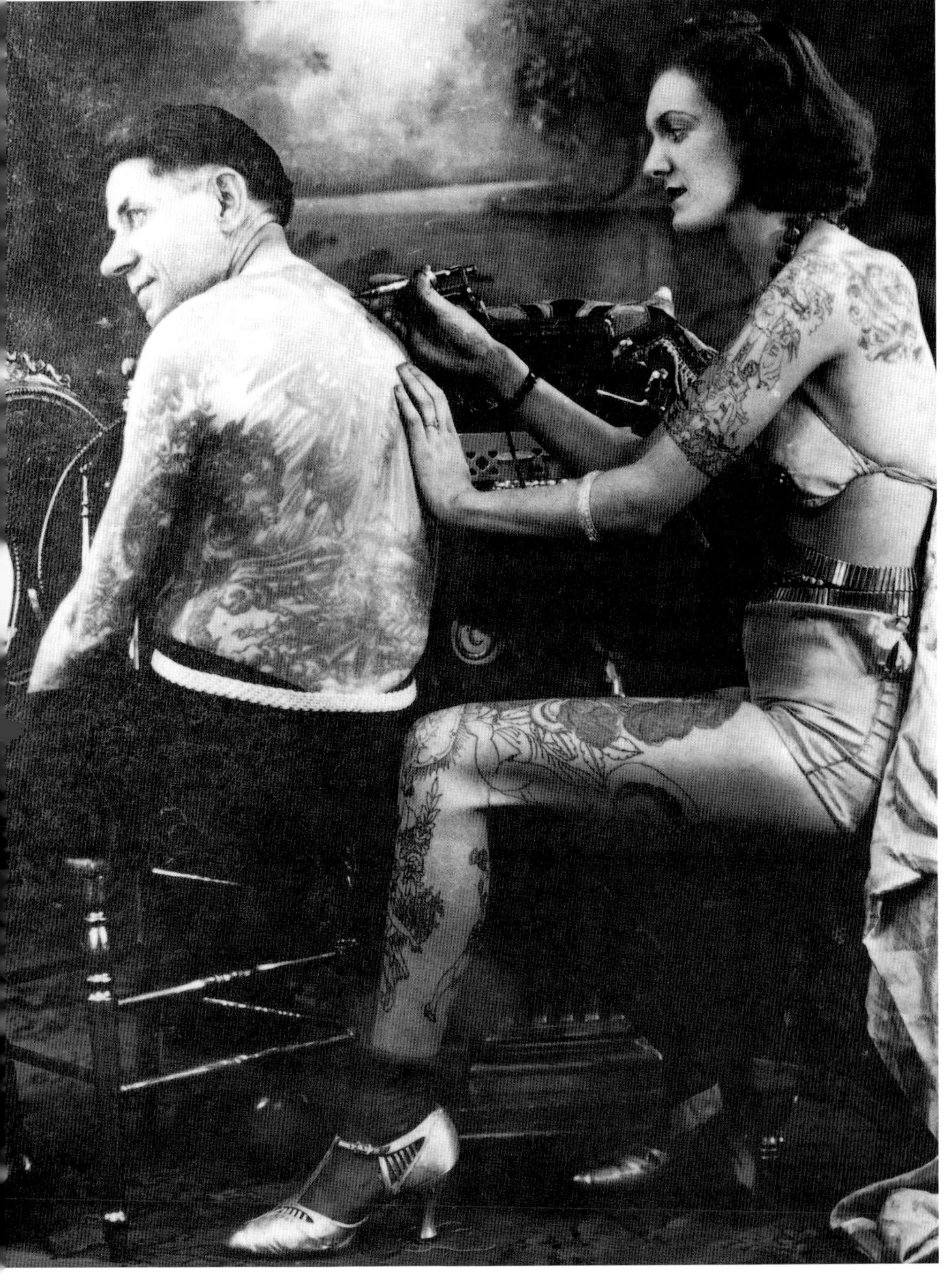

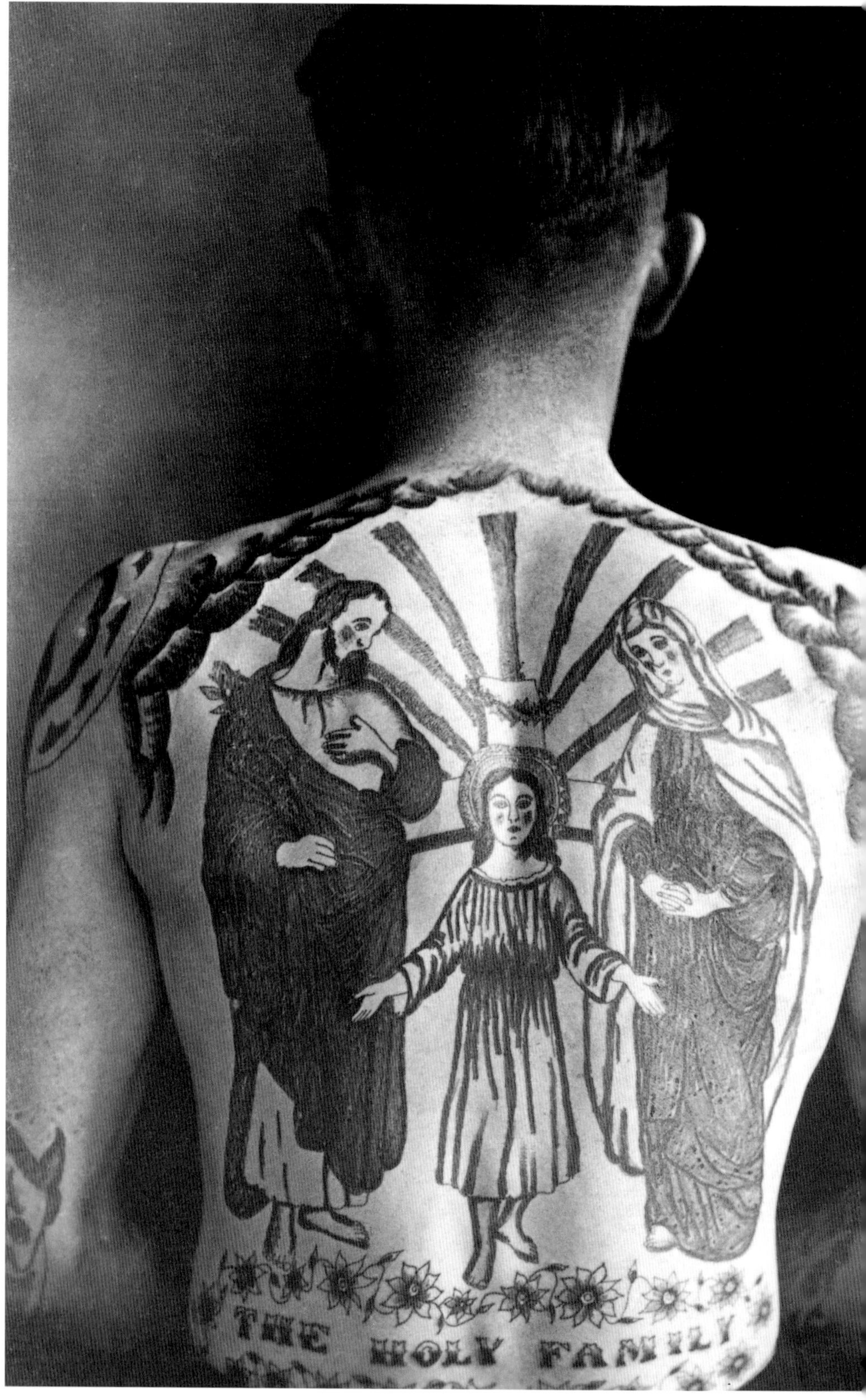
THE HOLY FAMILY

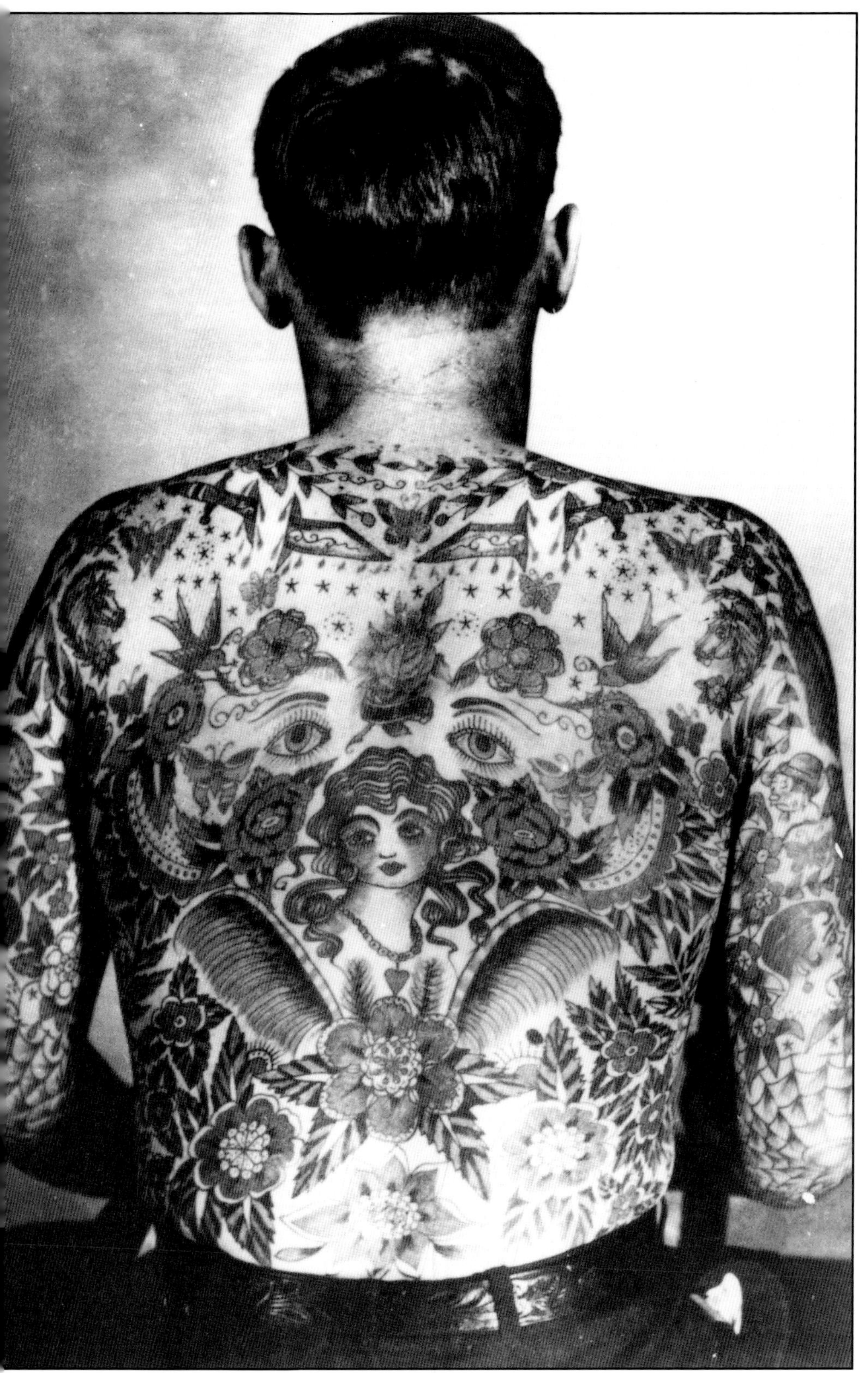

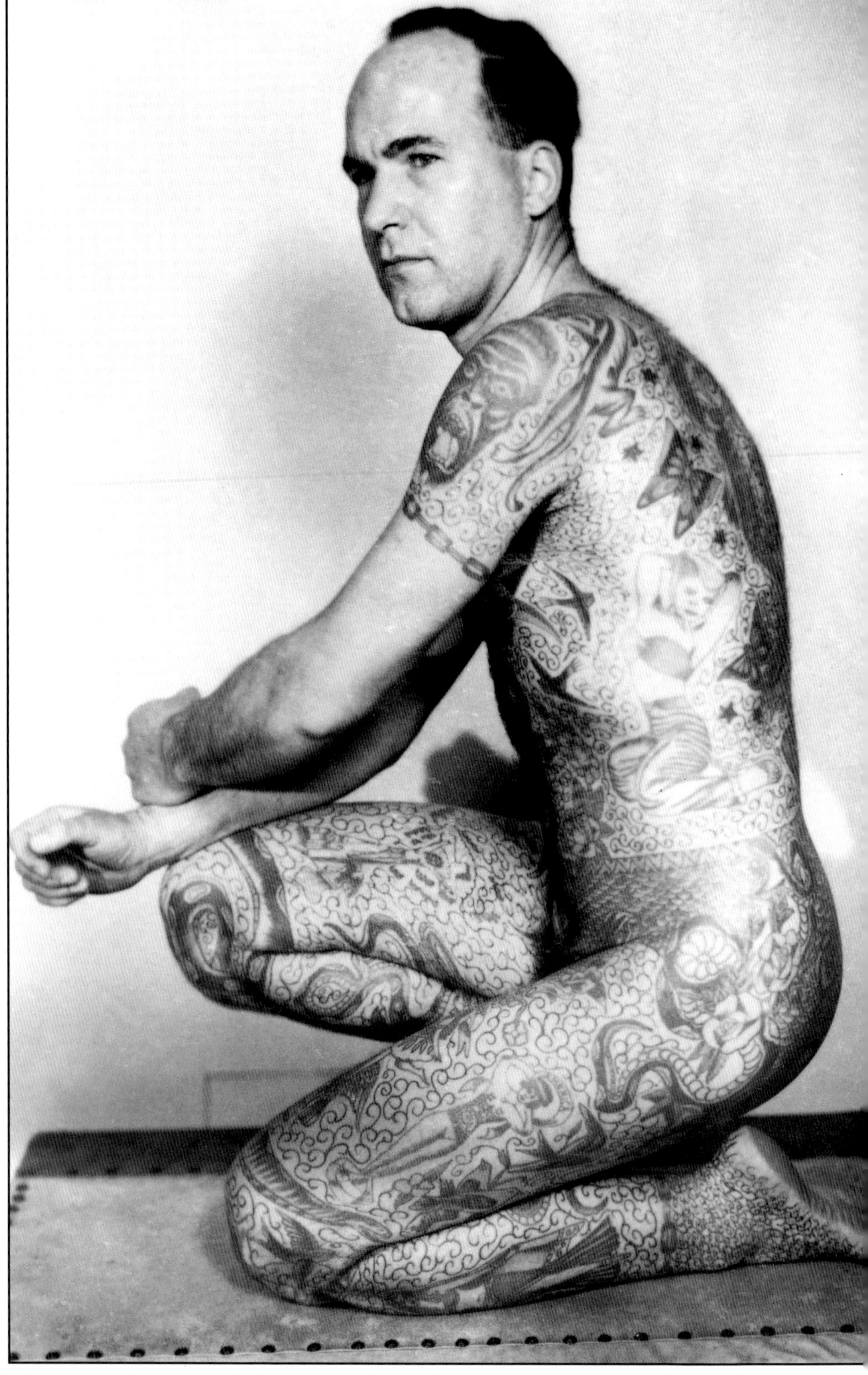

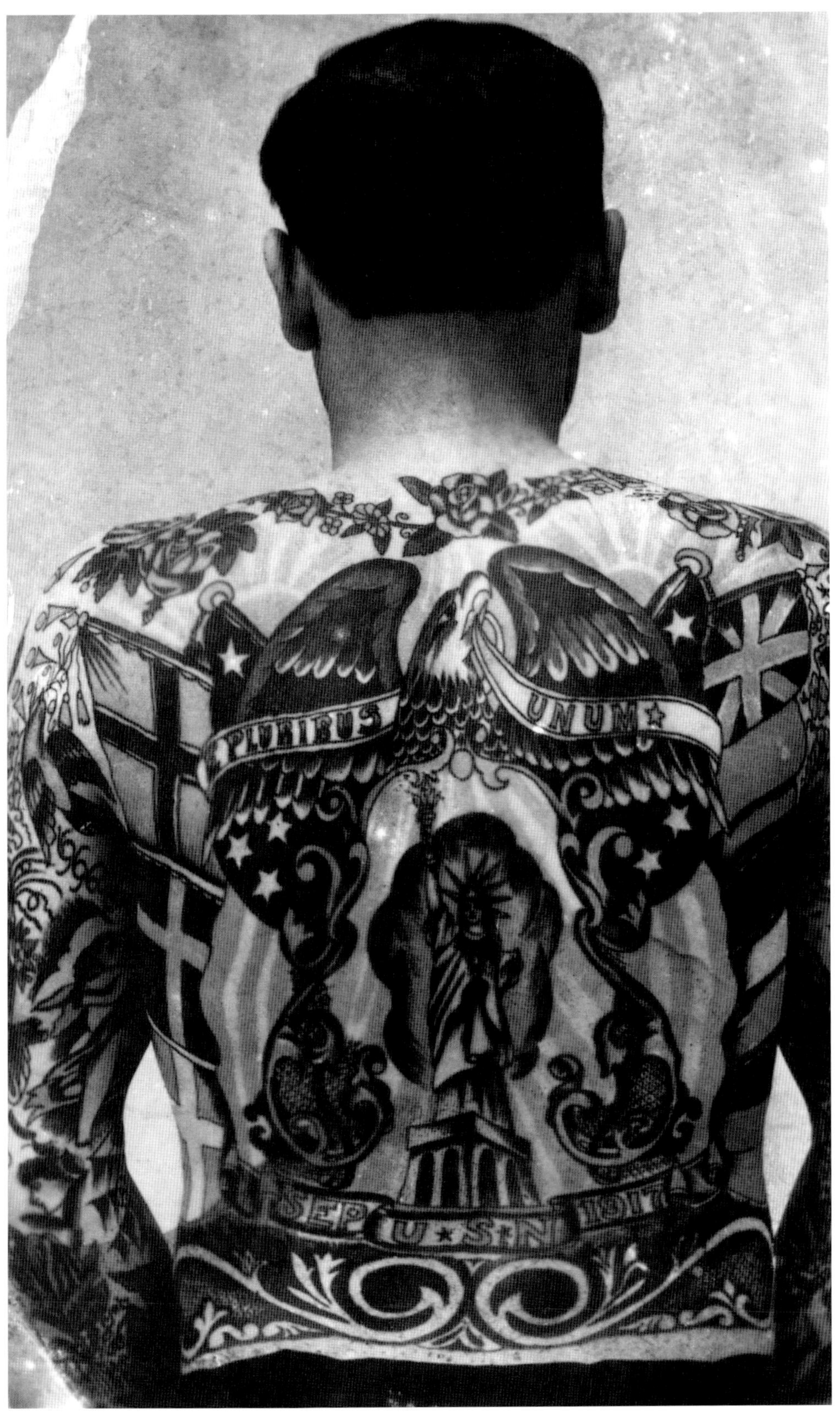

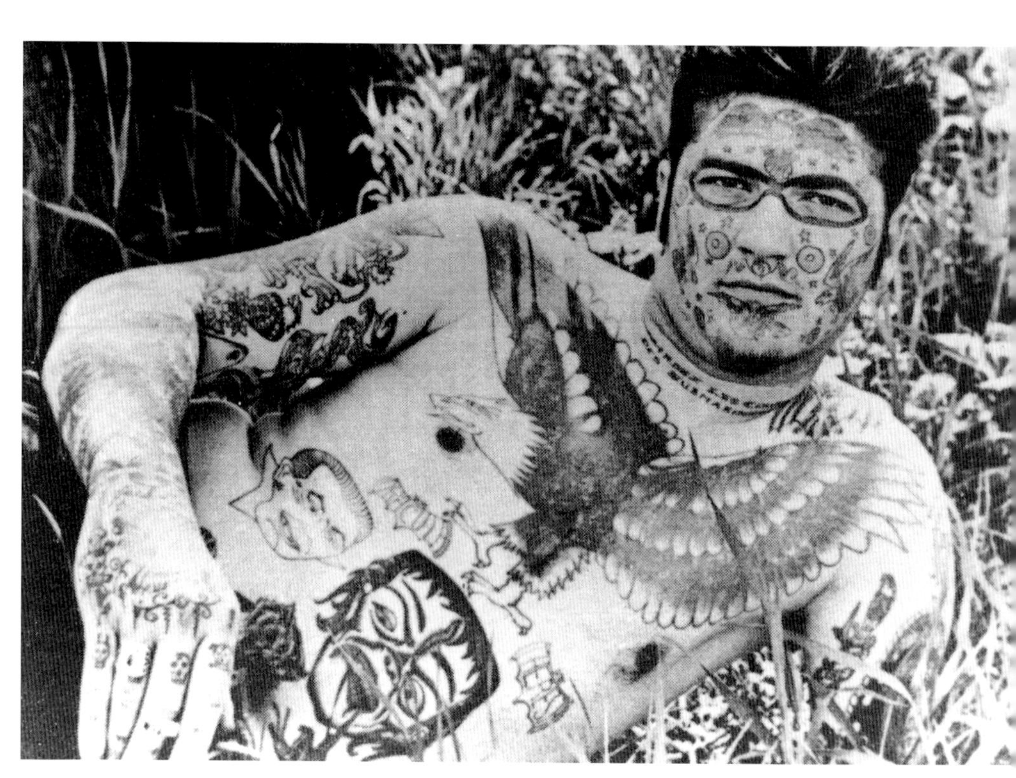

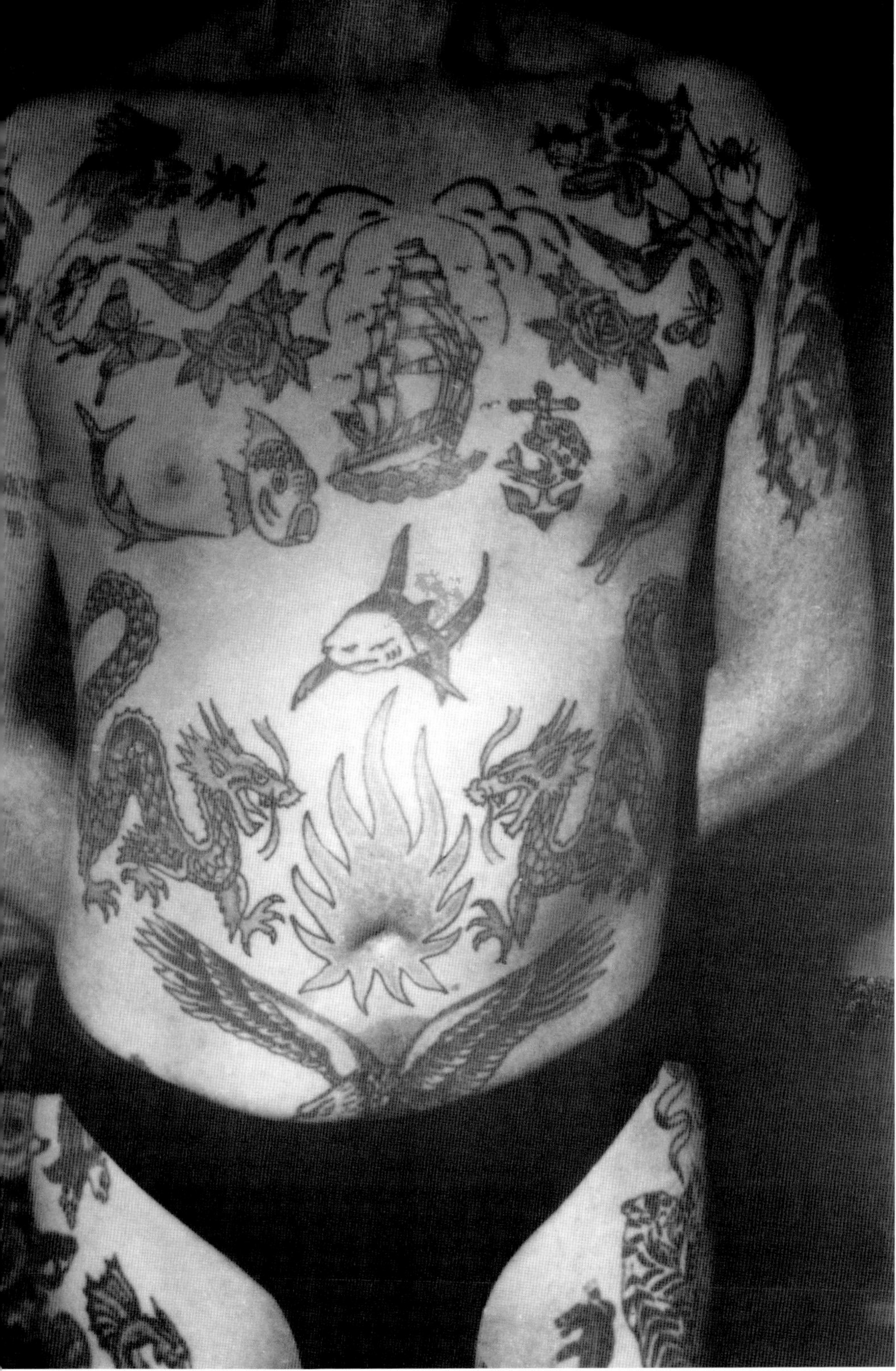

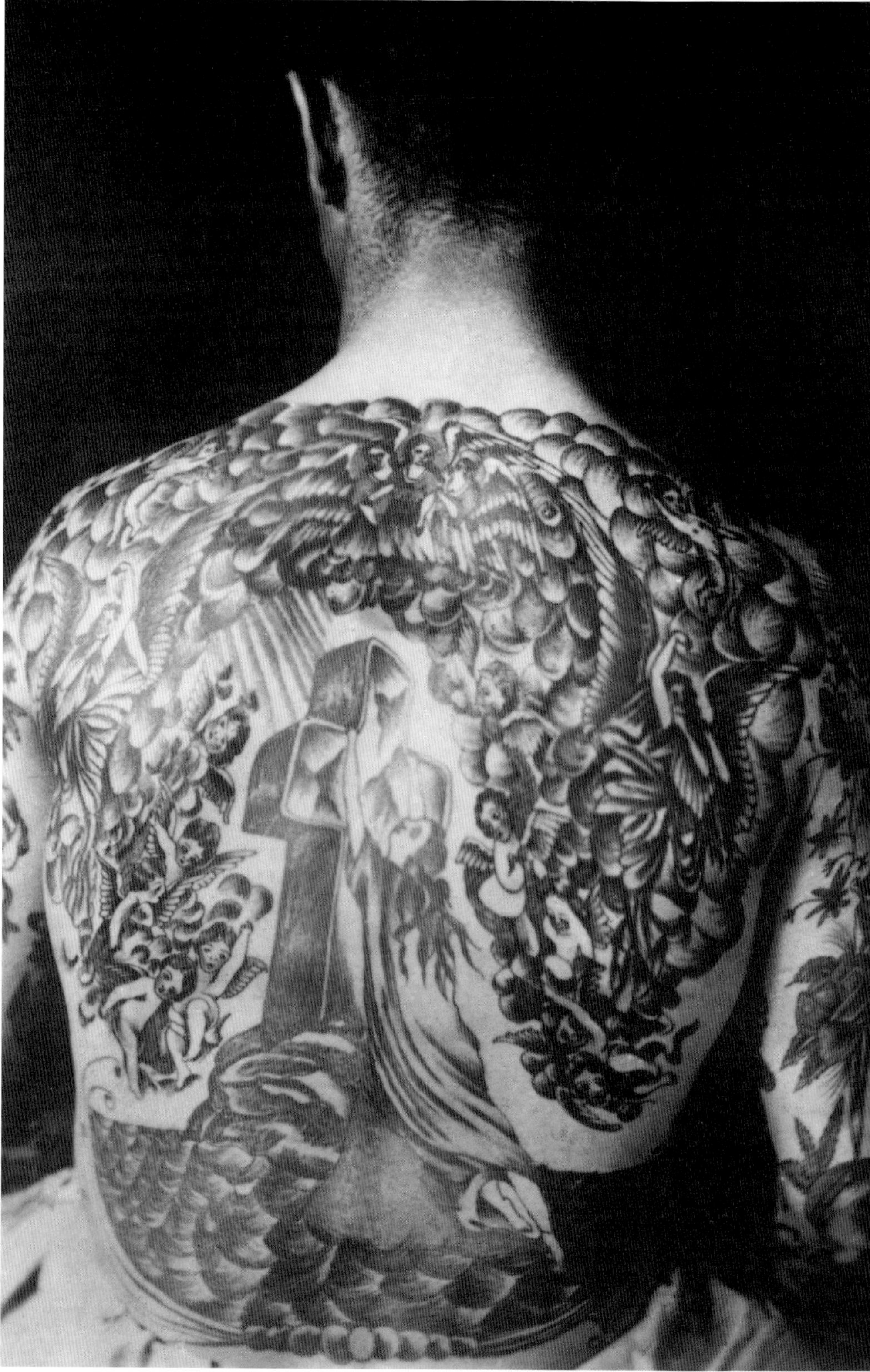

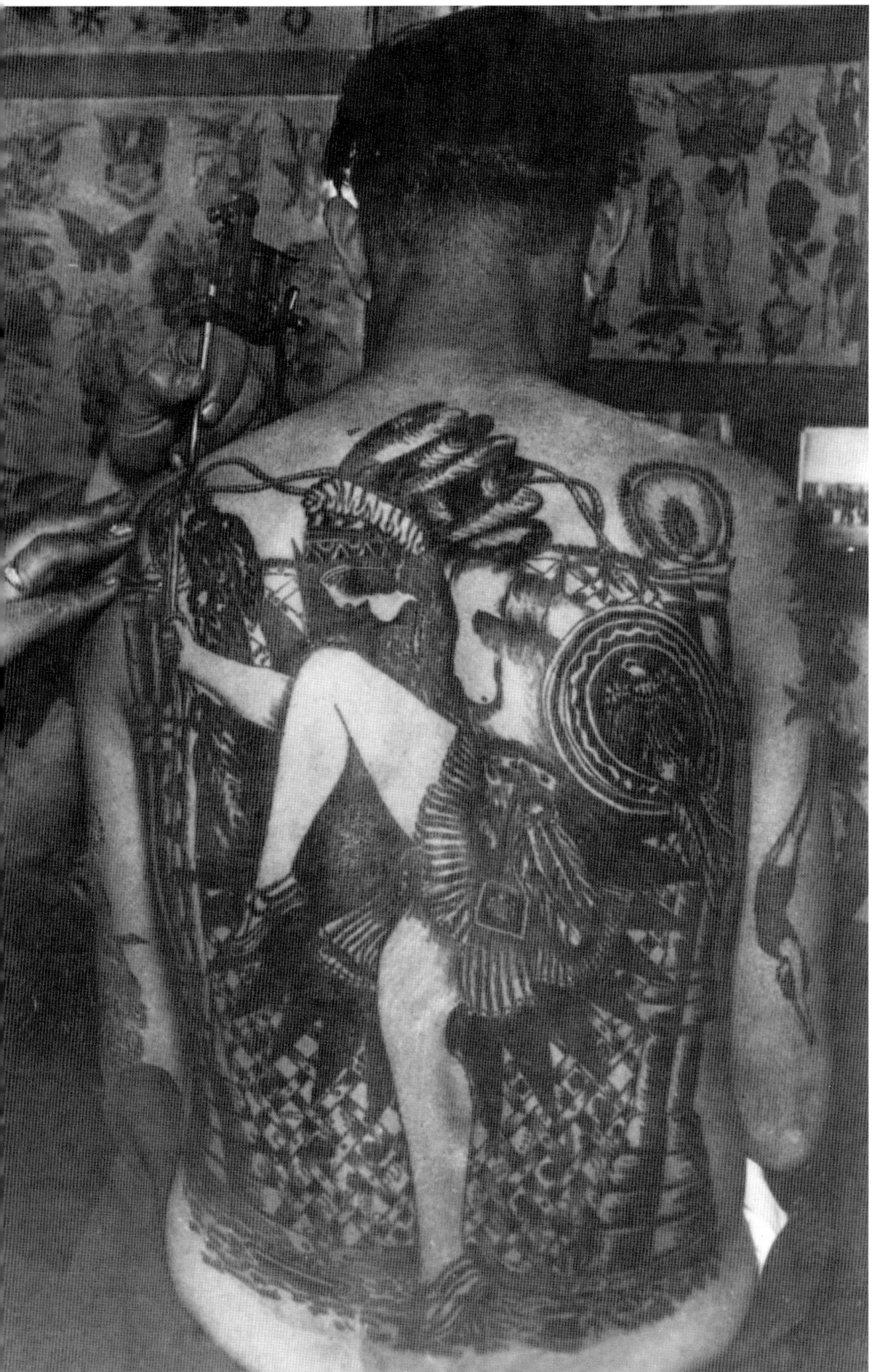

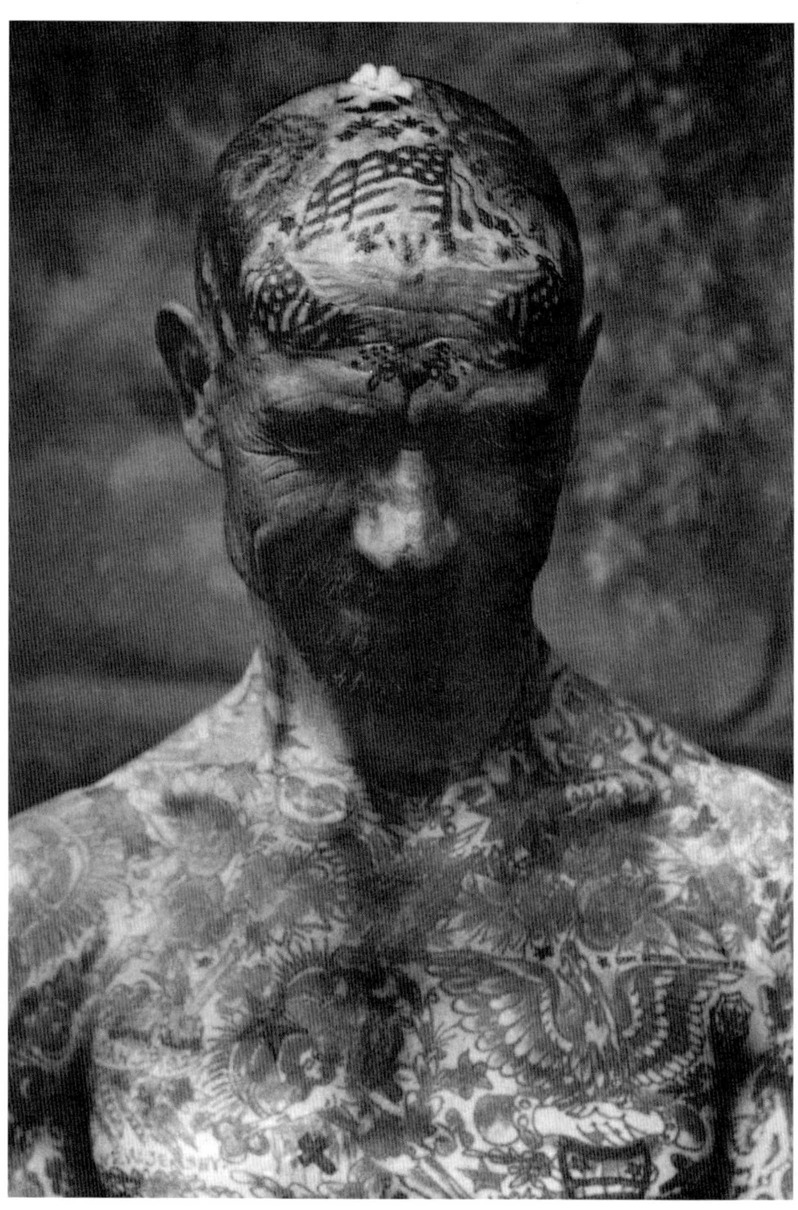

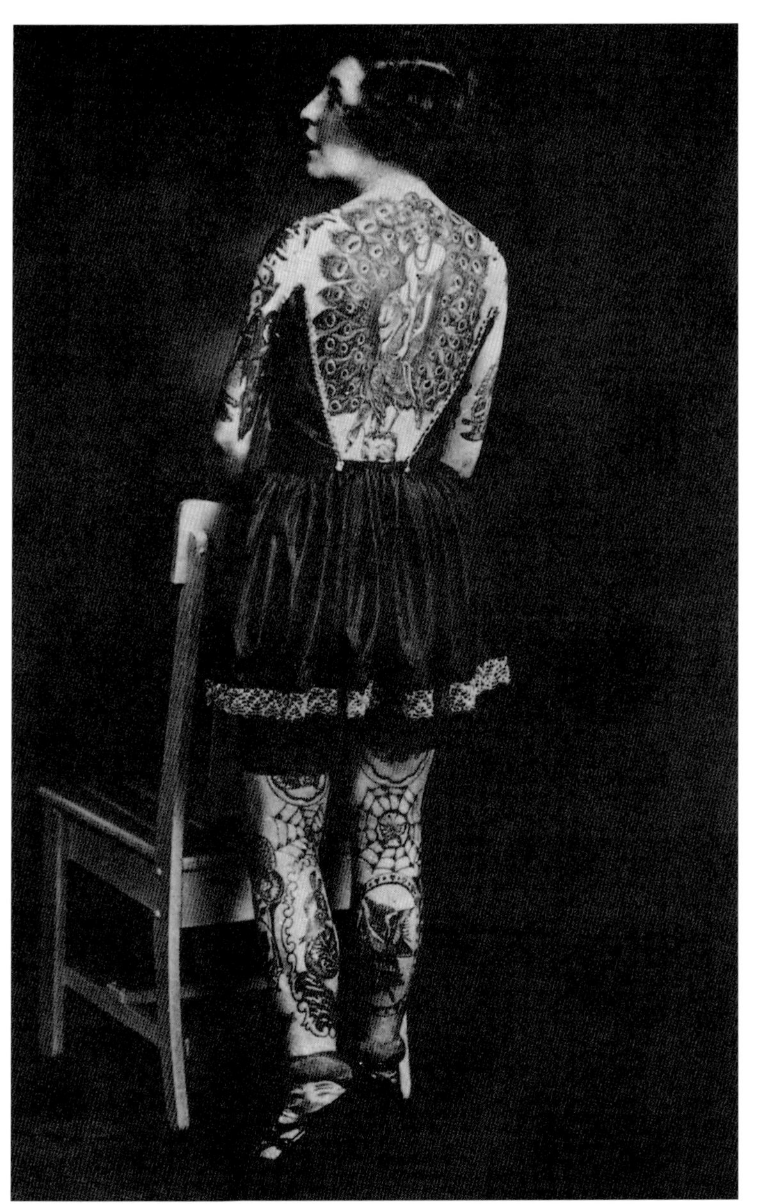

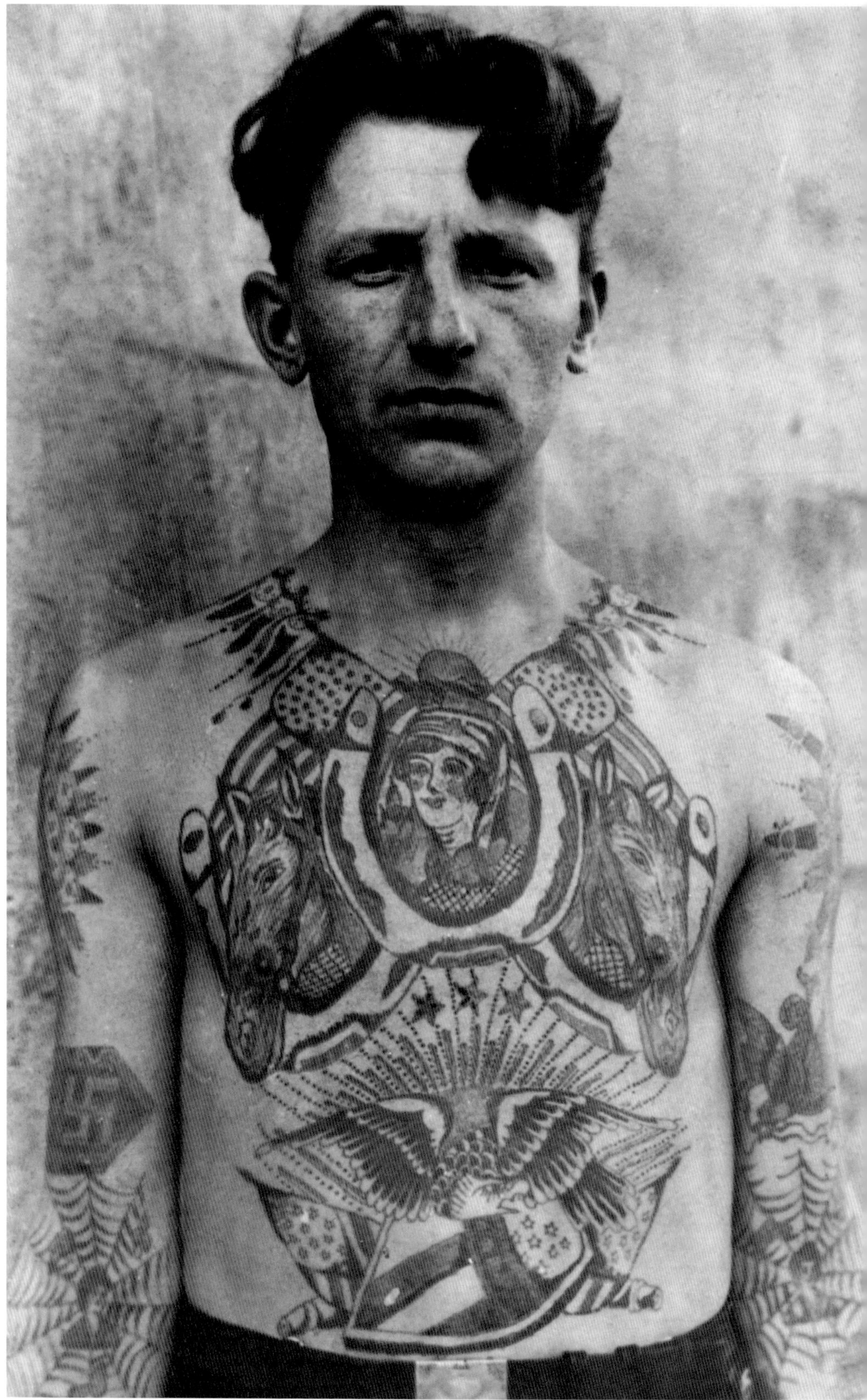

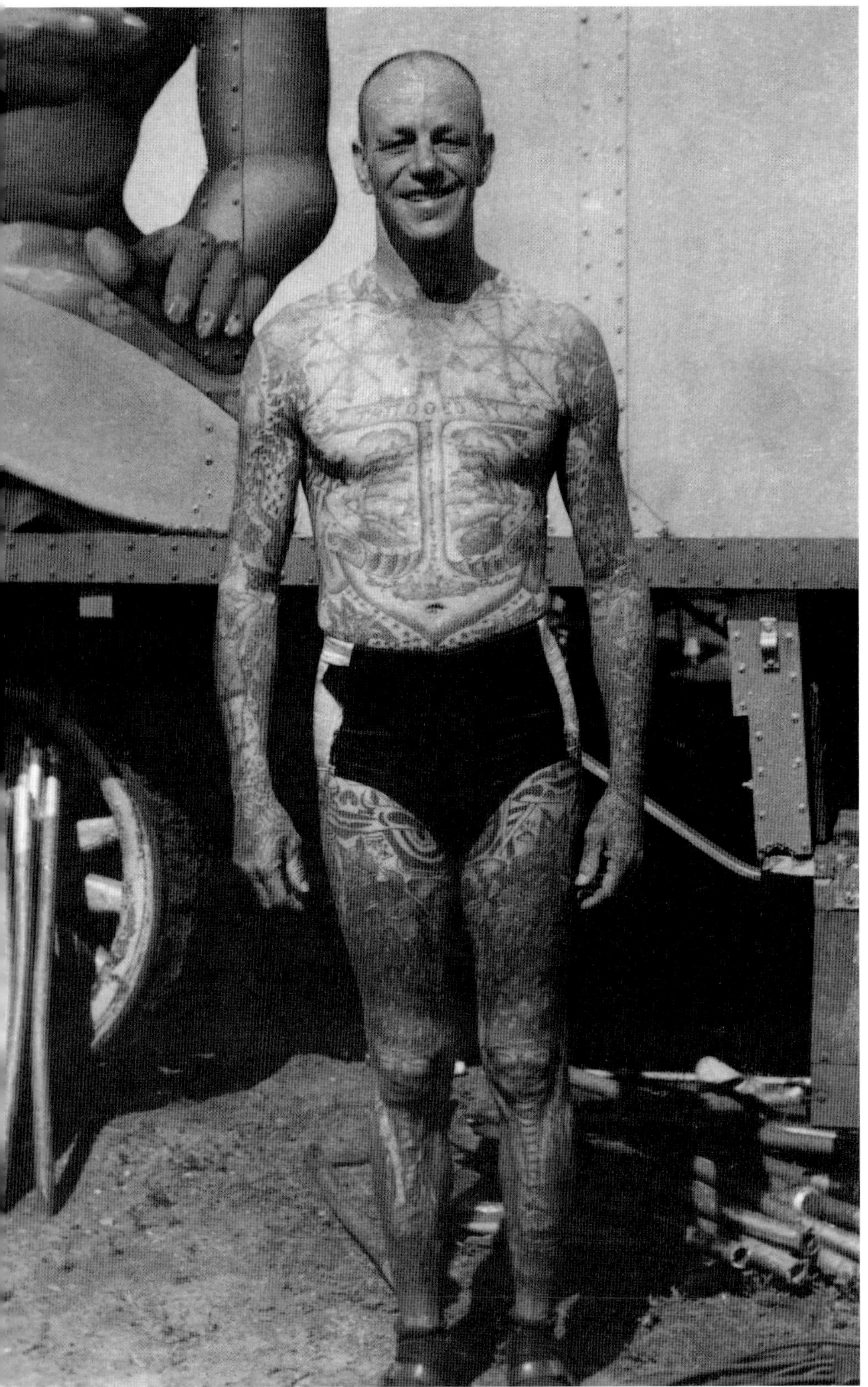

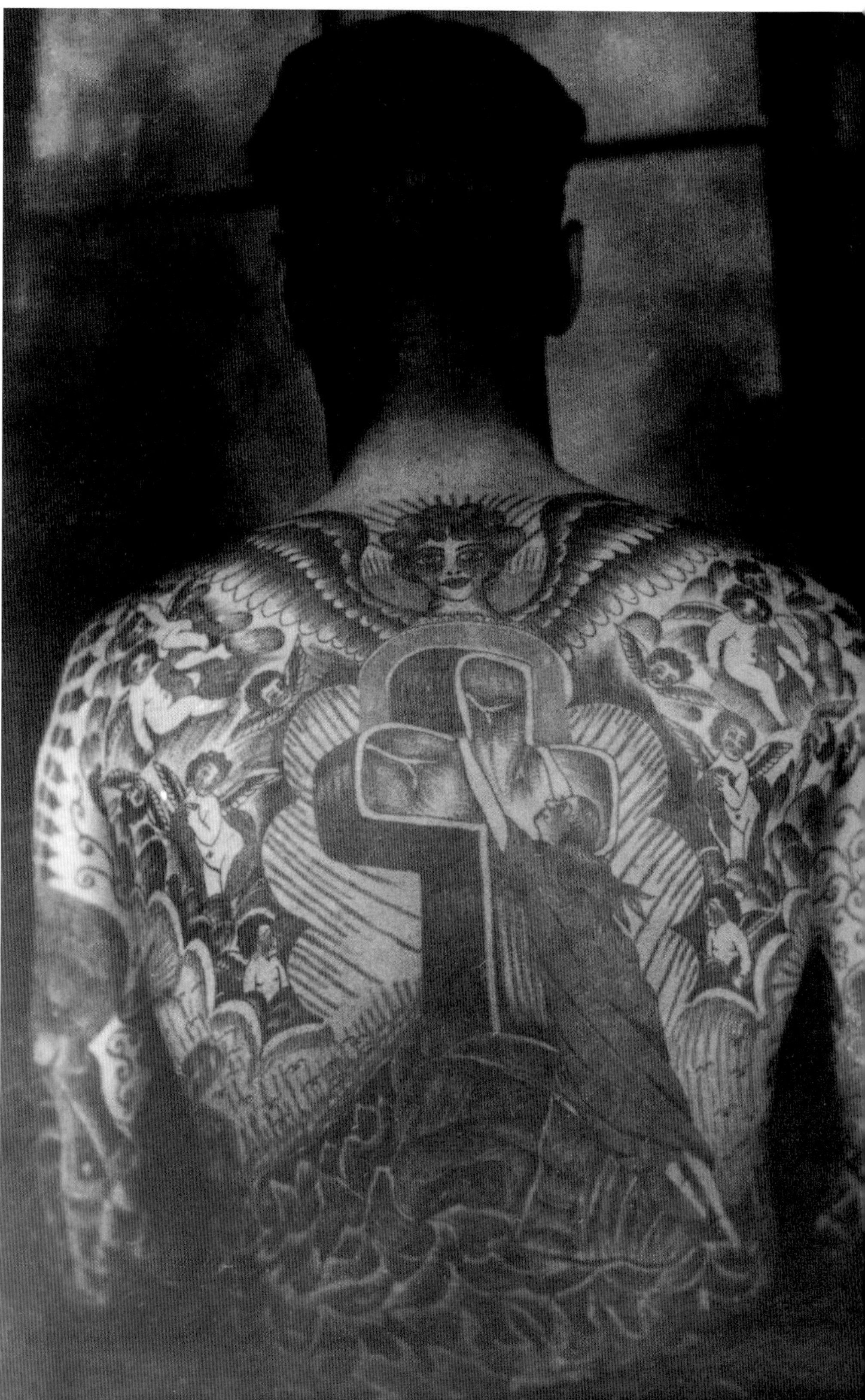

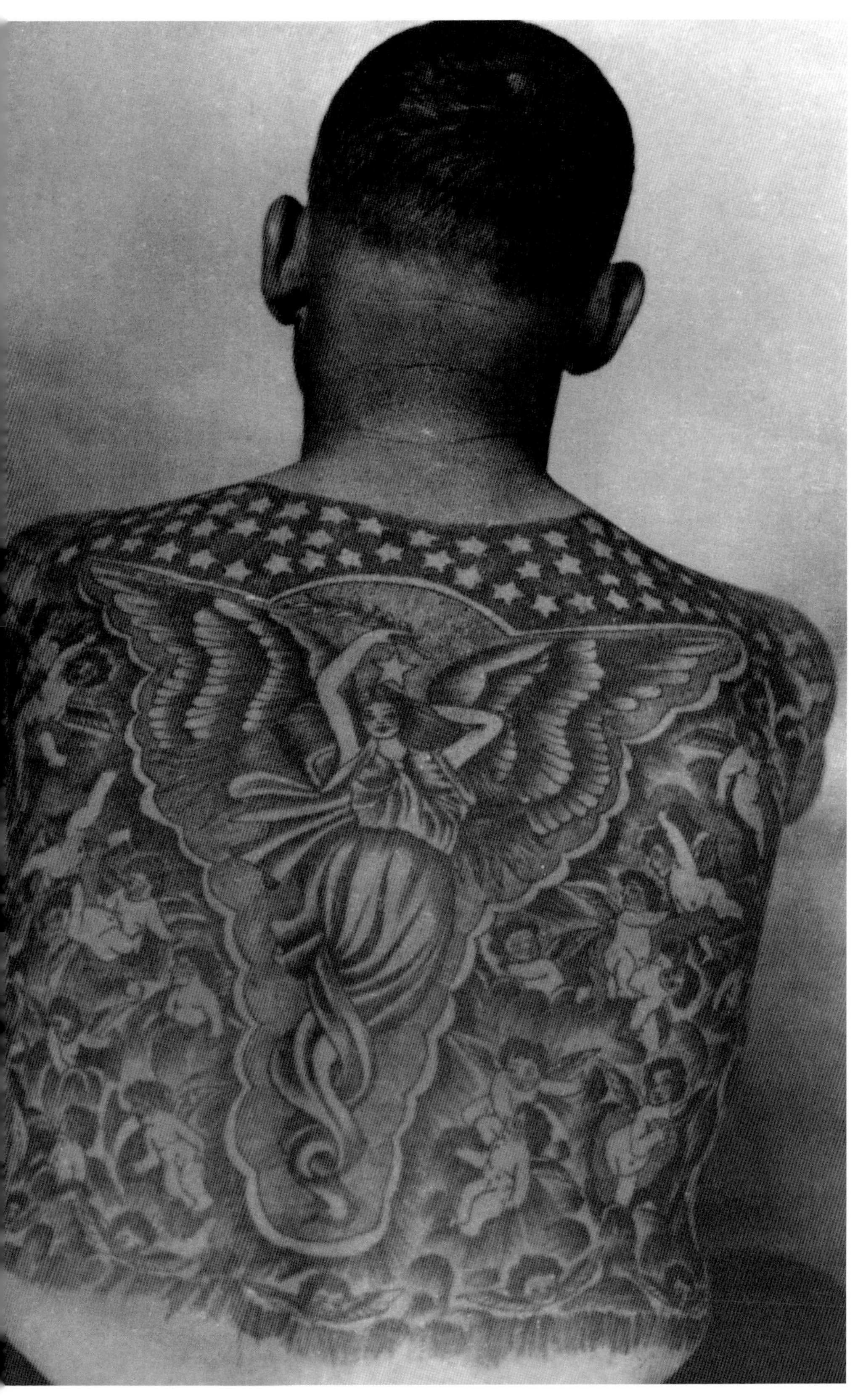

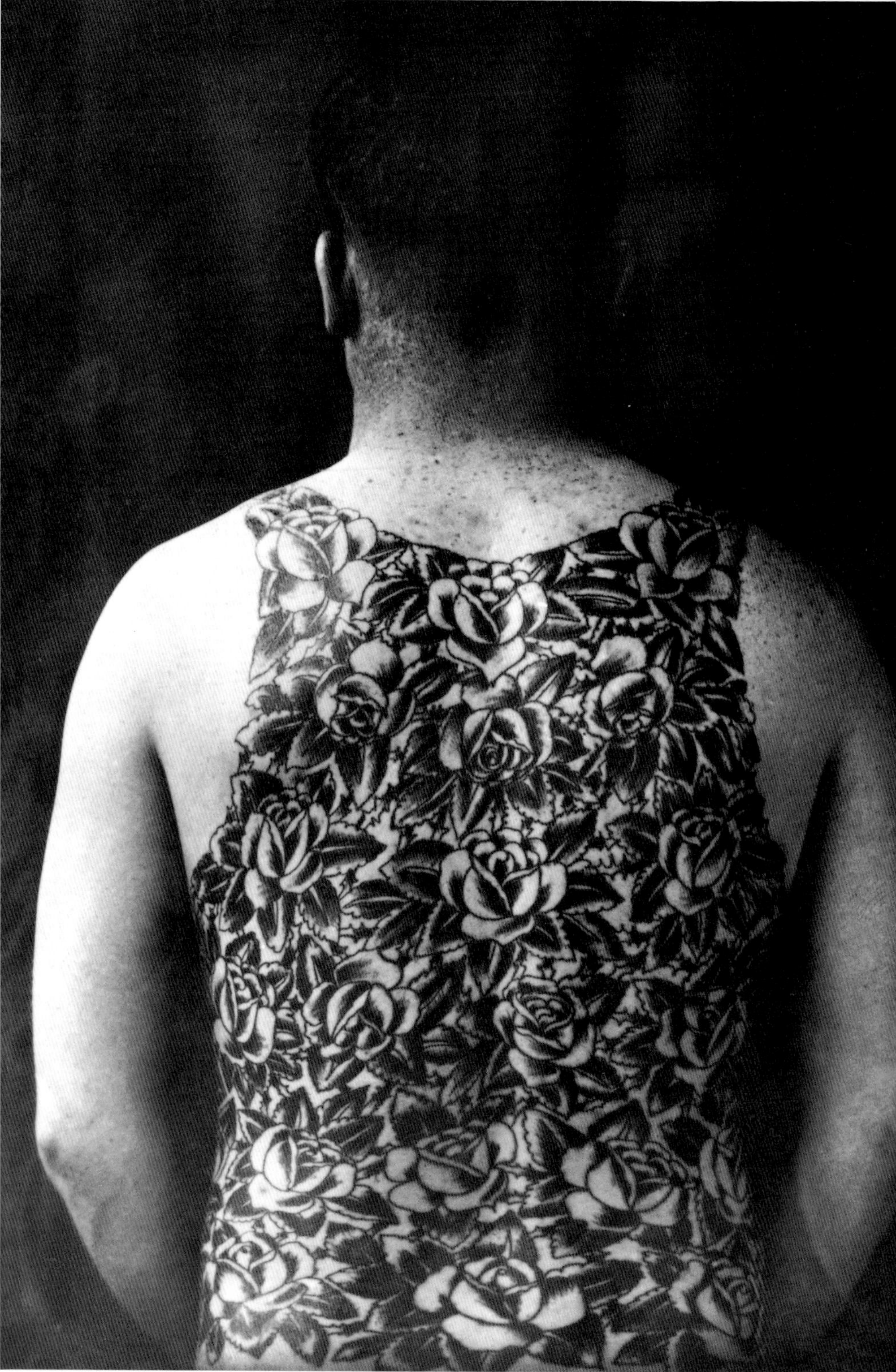

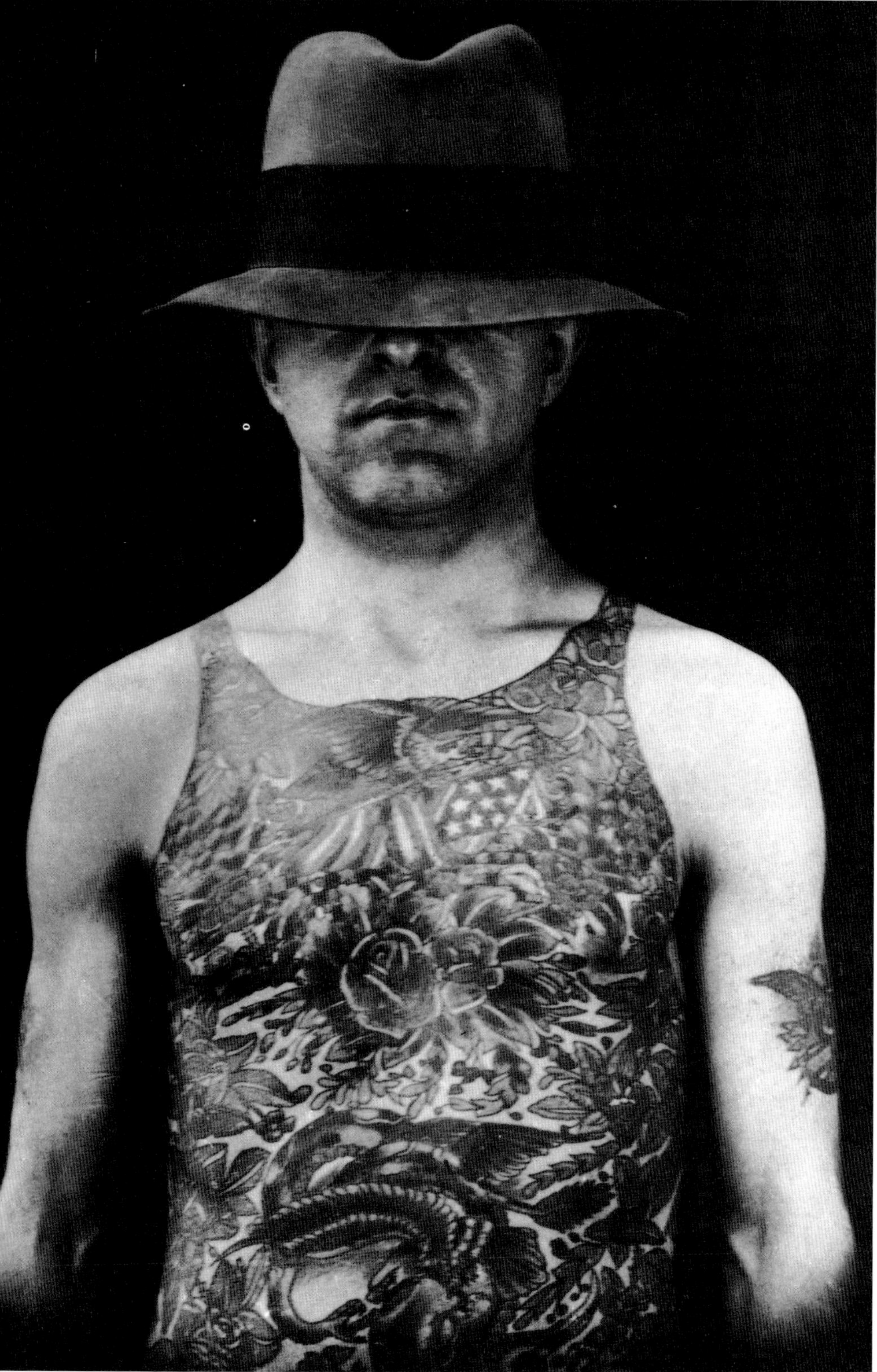

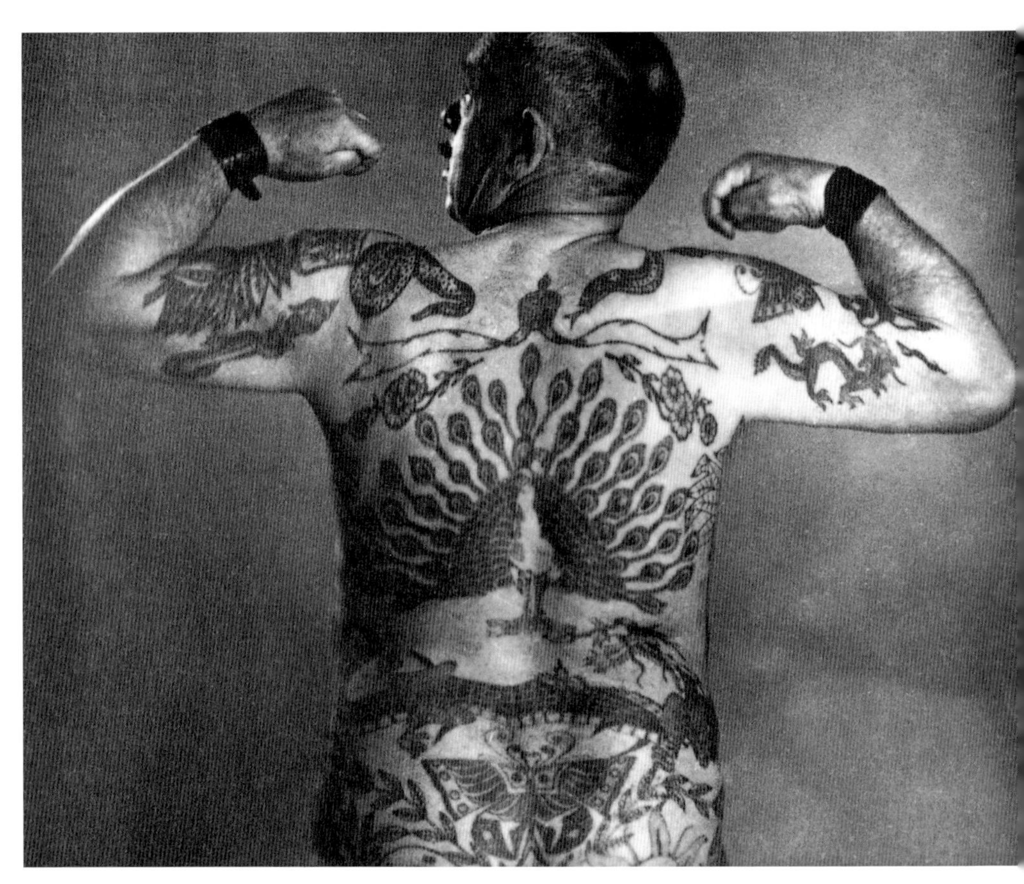

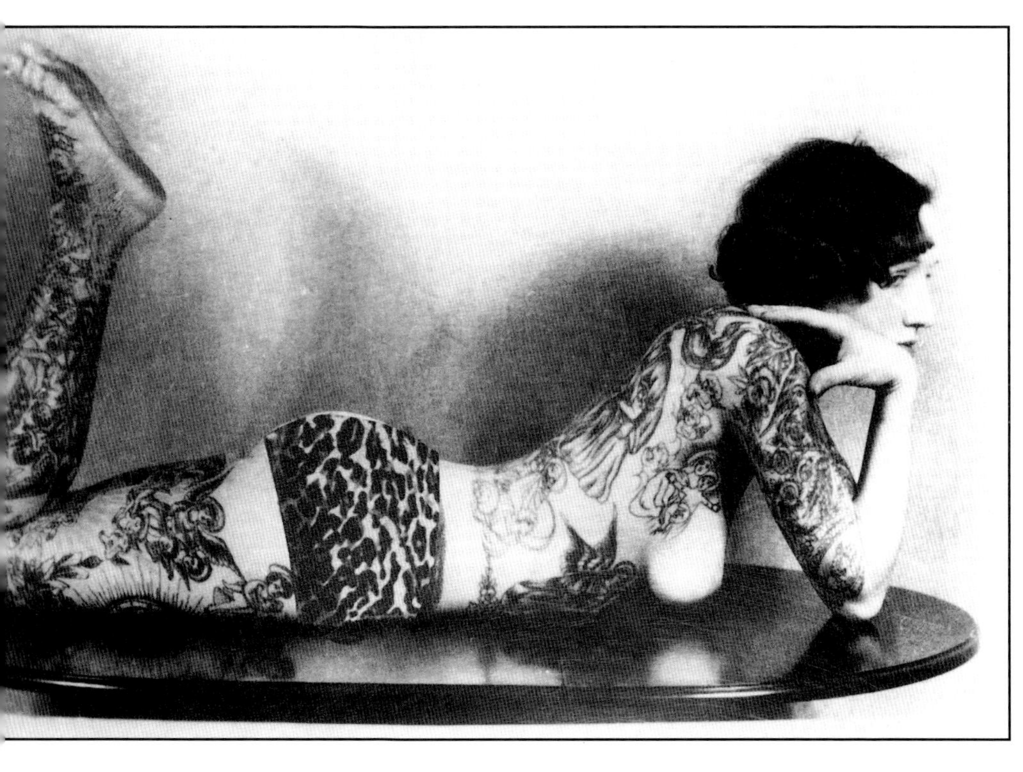

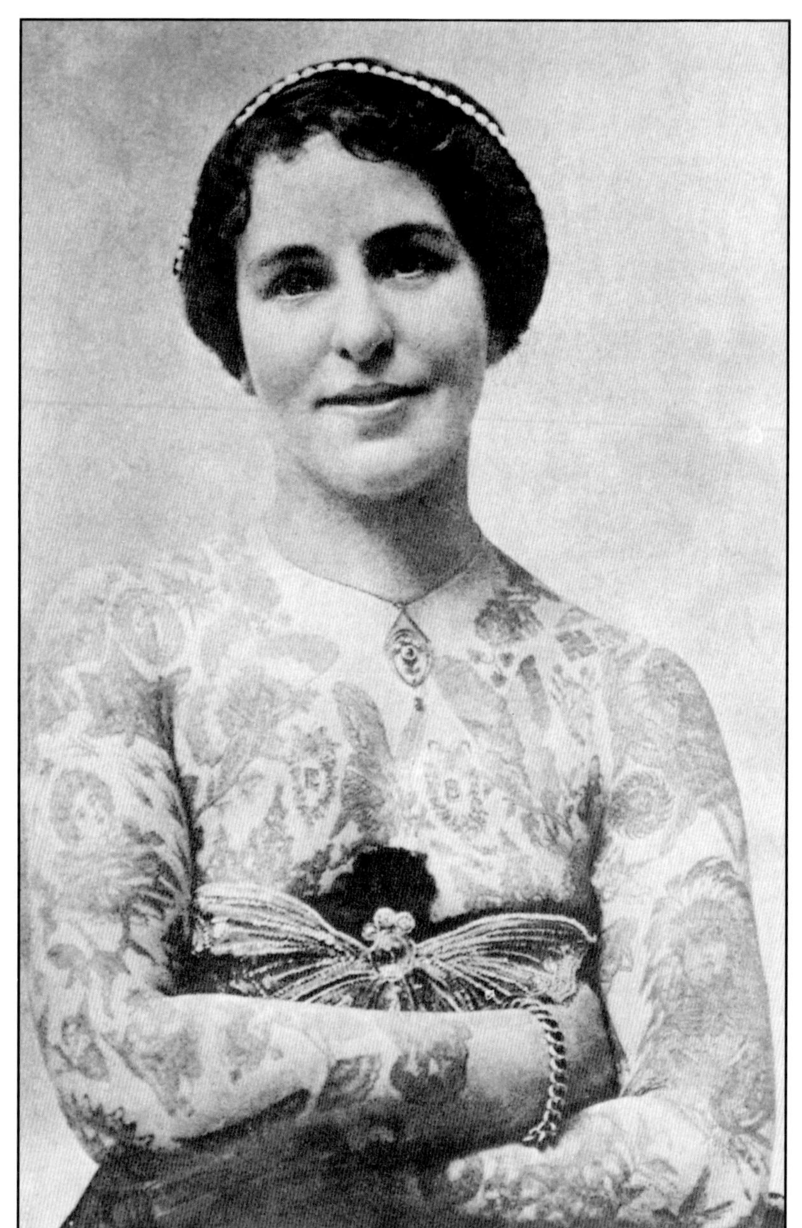

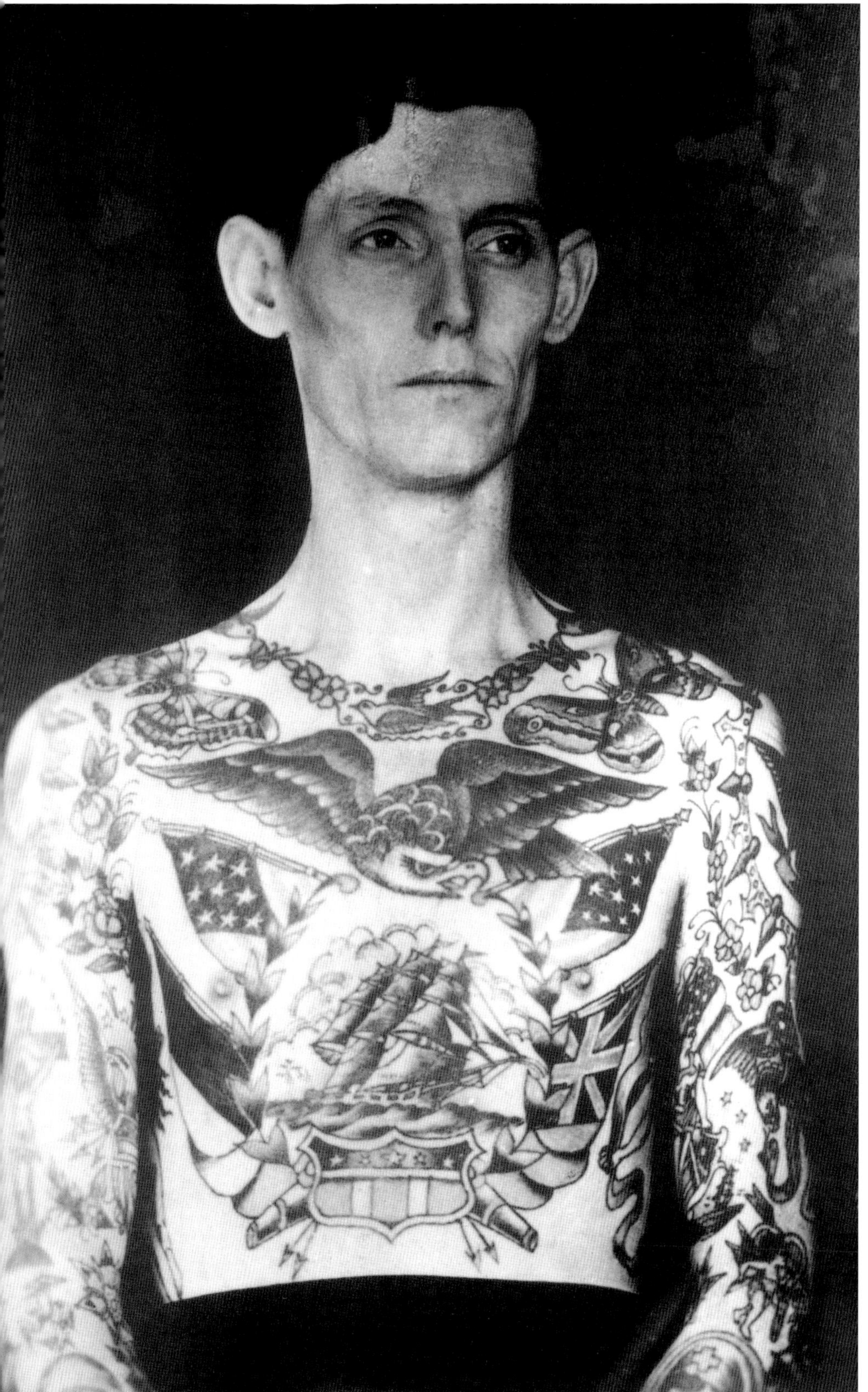

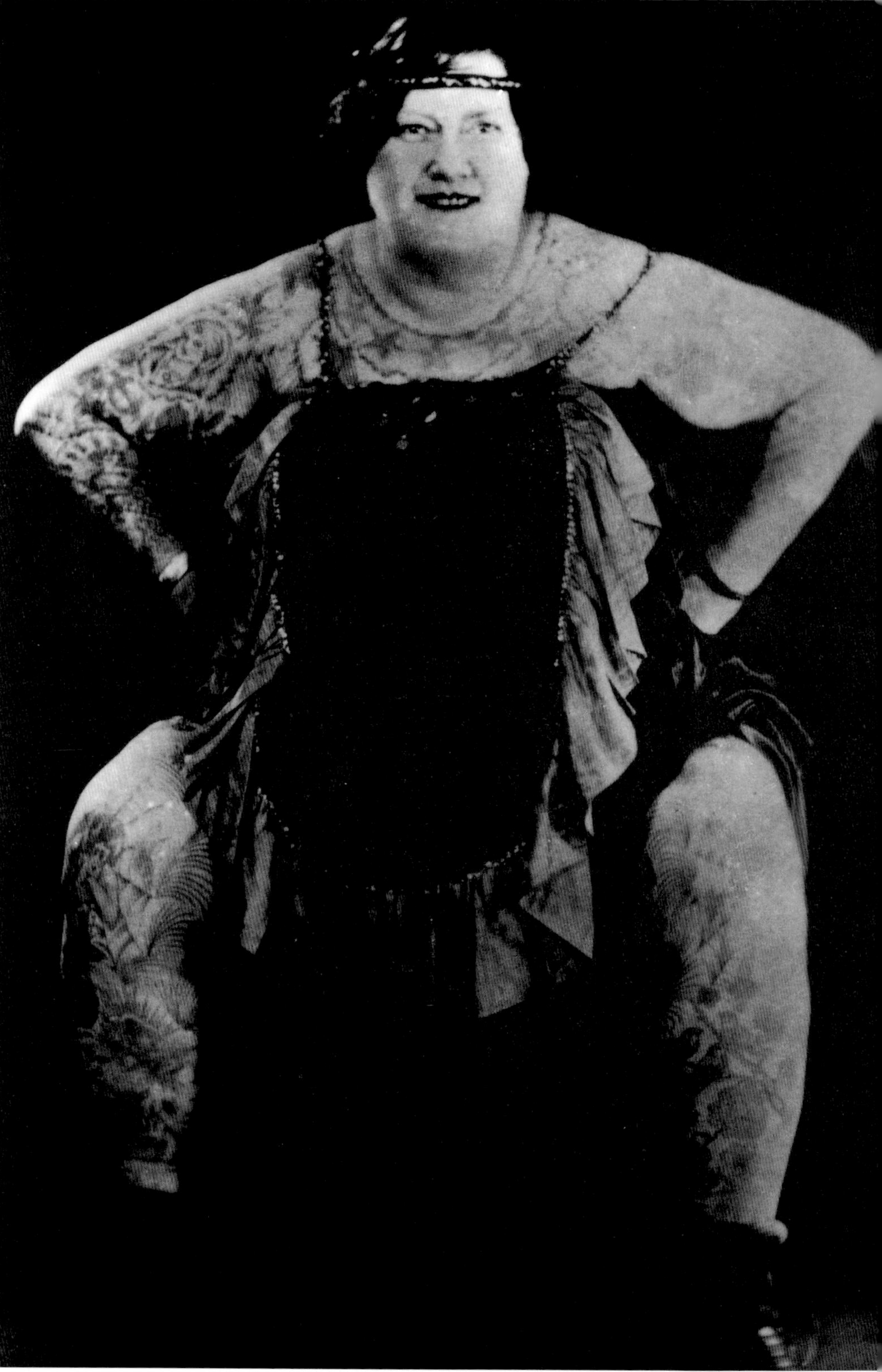

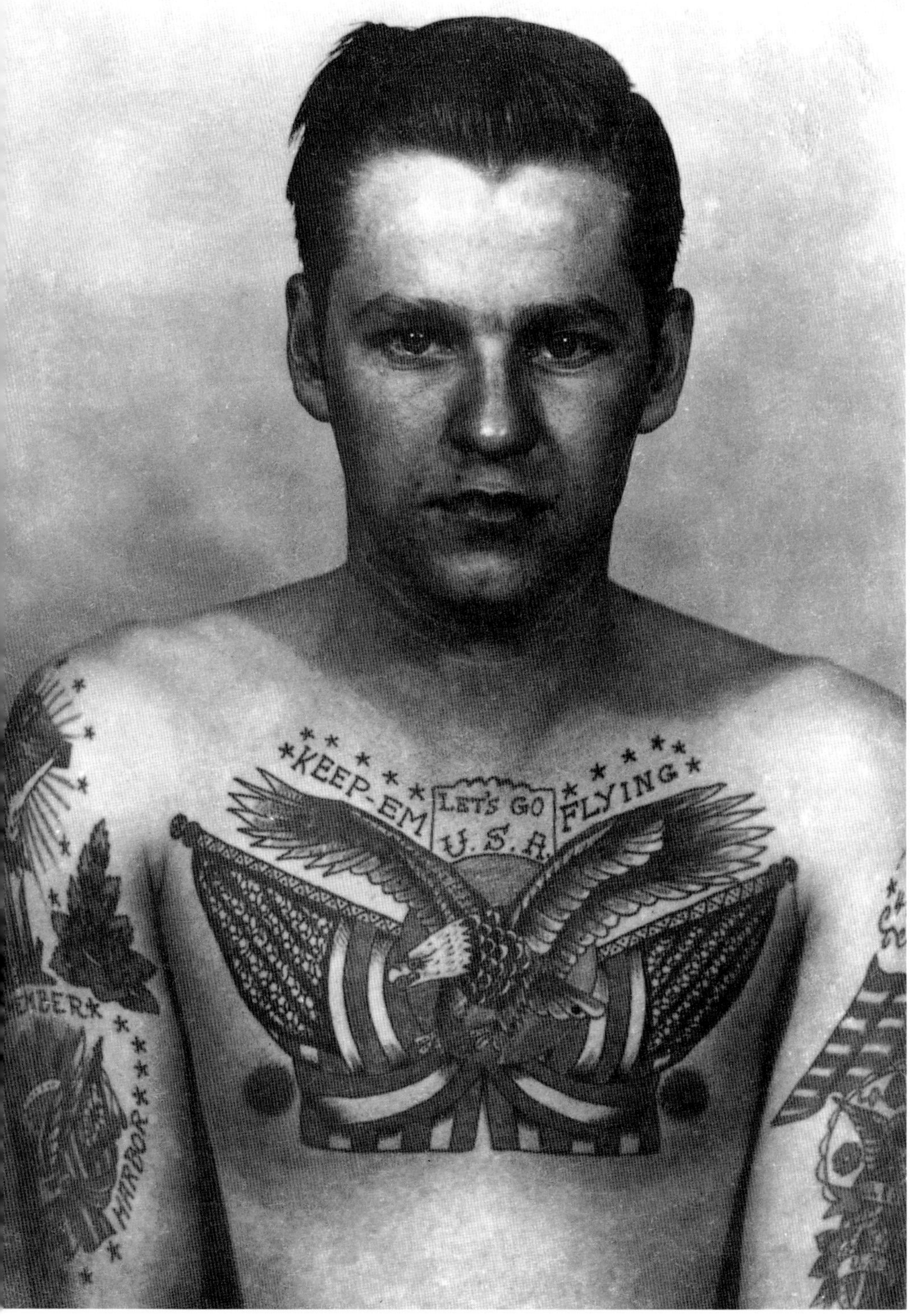

*KEEP-EM
LETS GO
U.S.A.
FLYING*
EMBER*
HARBOR

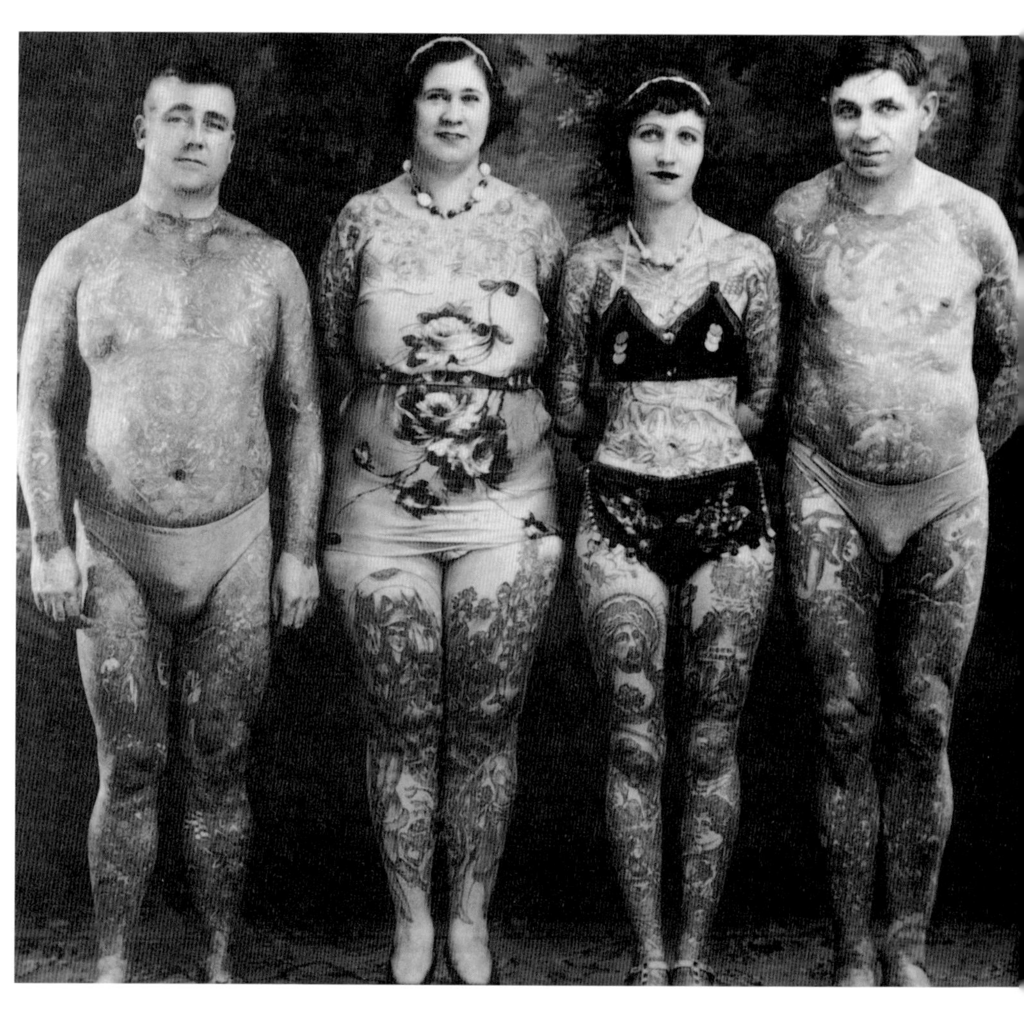

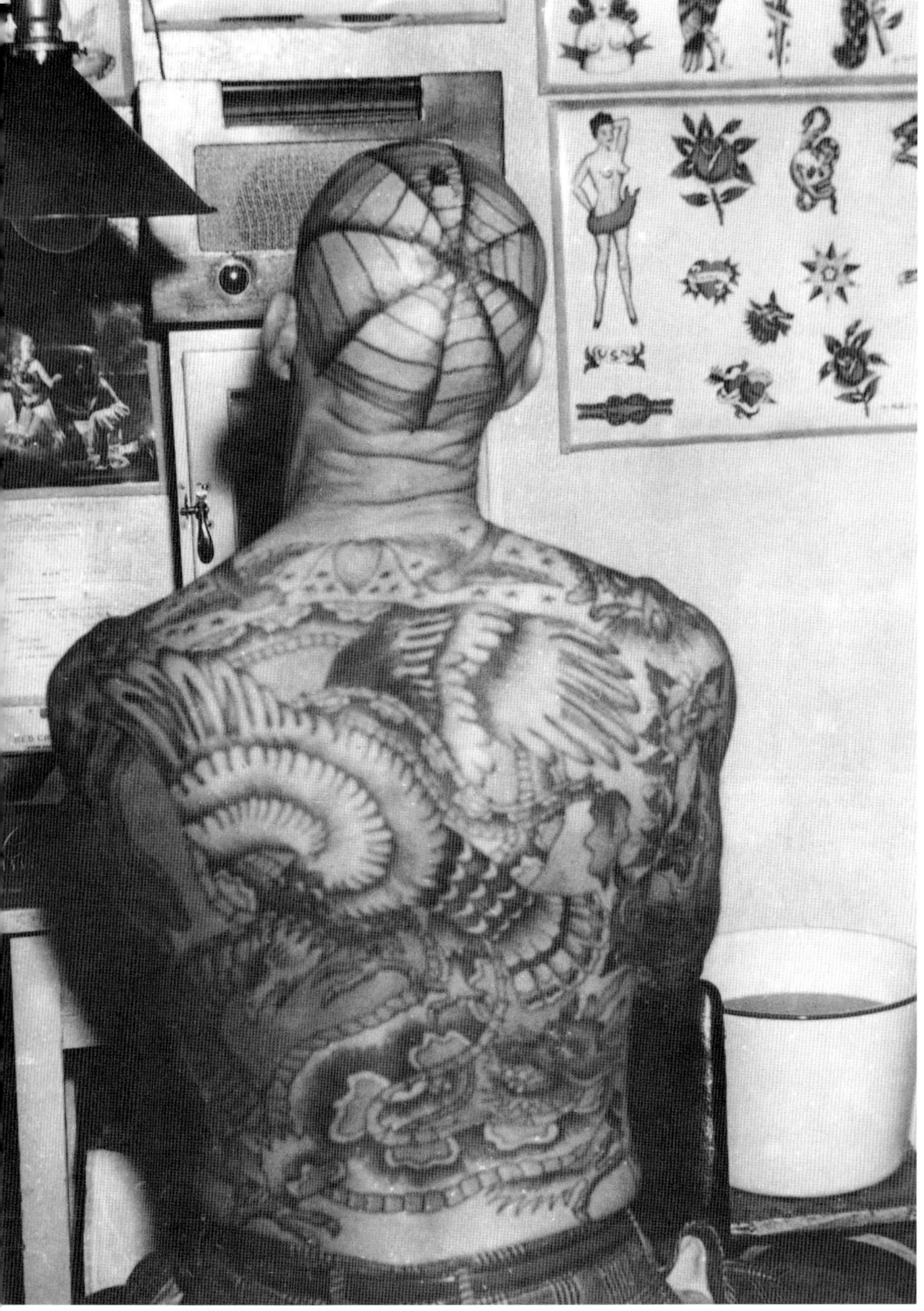

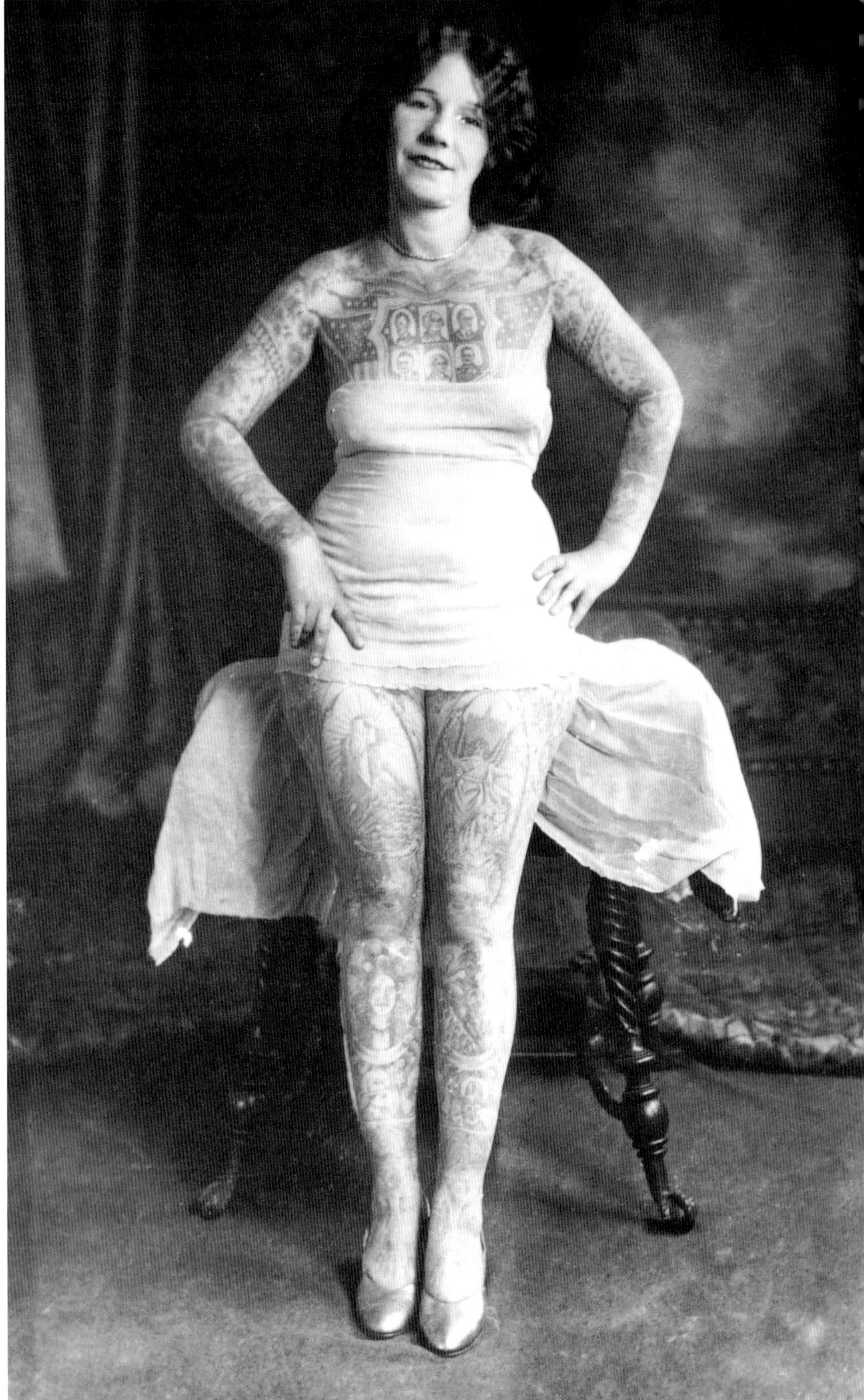

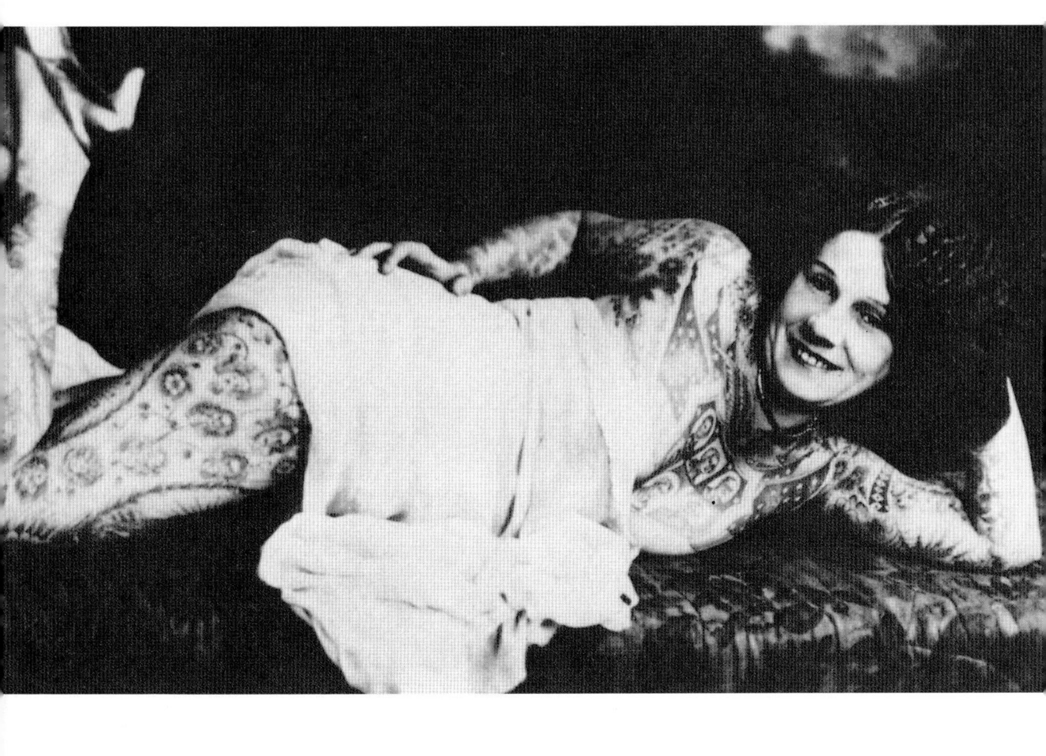

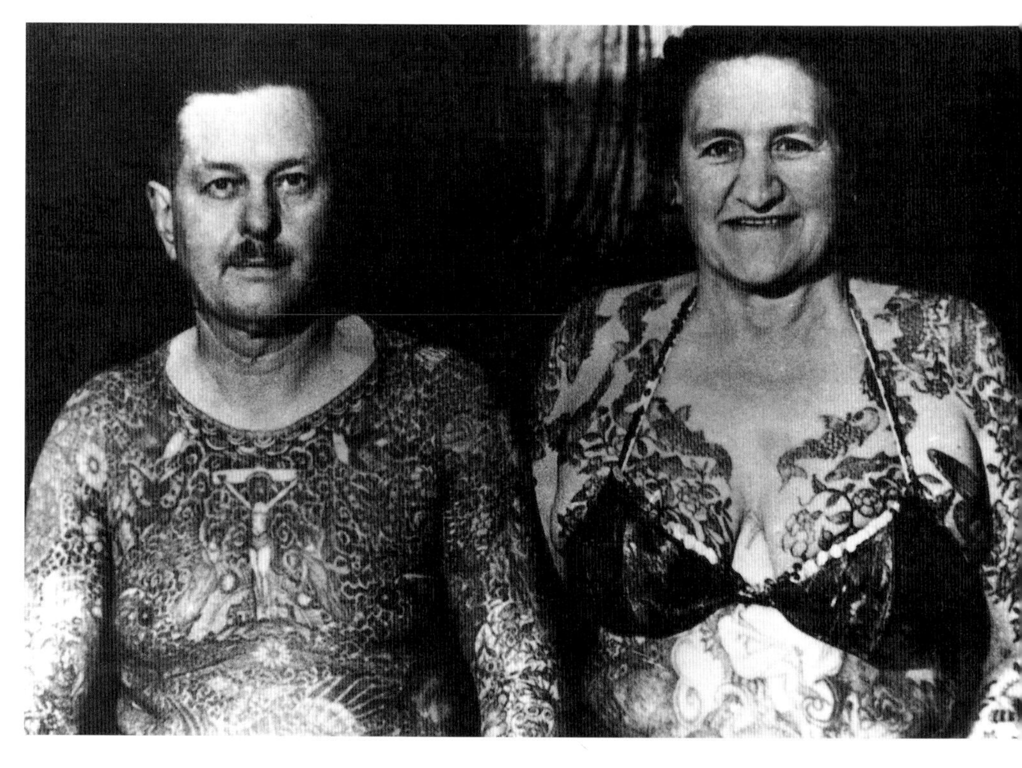

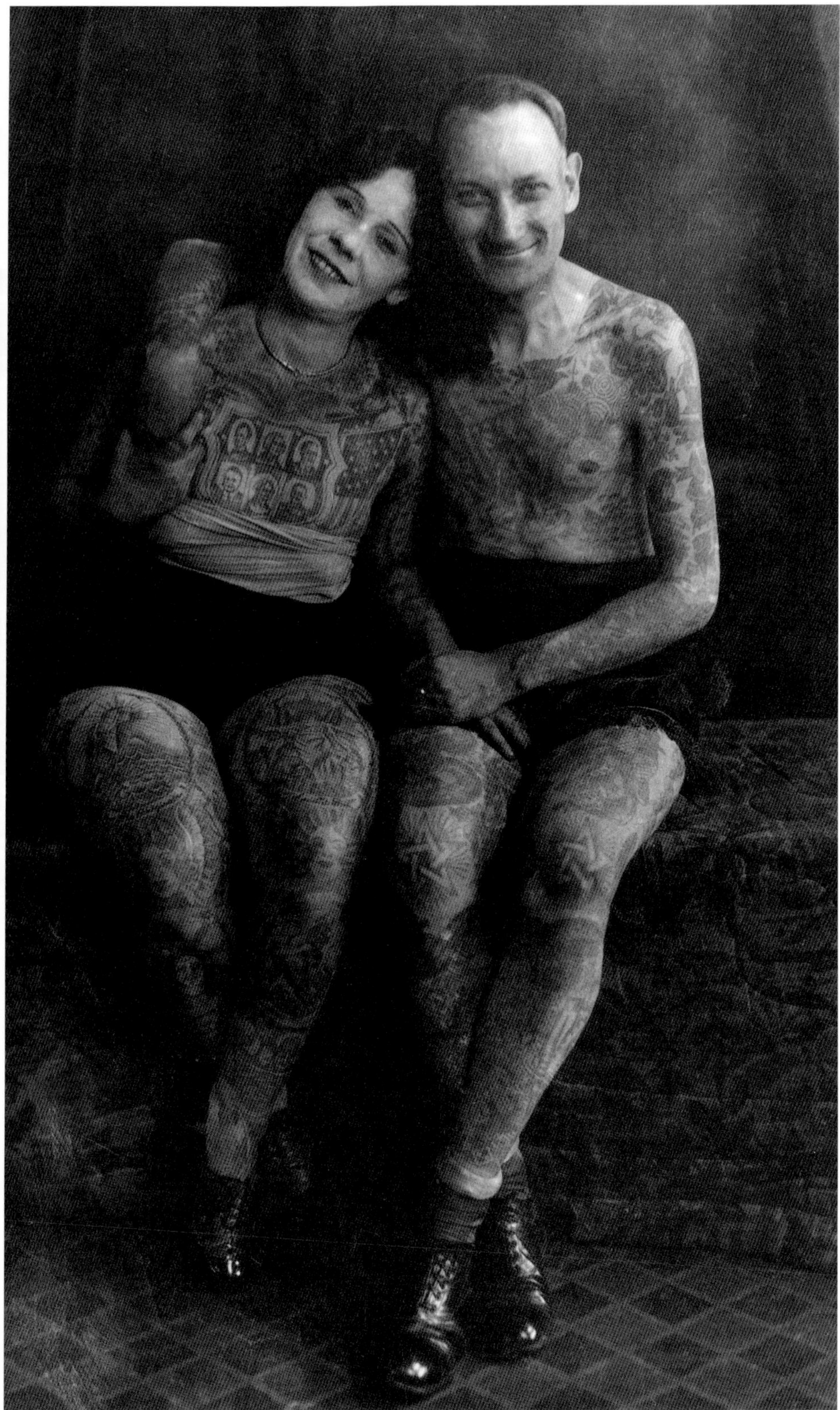

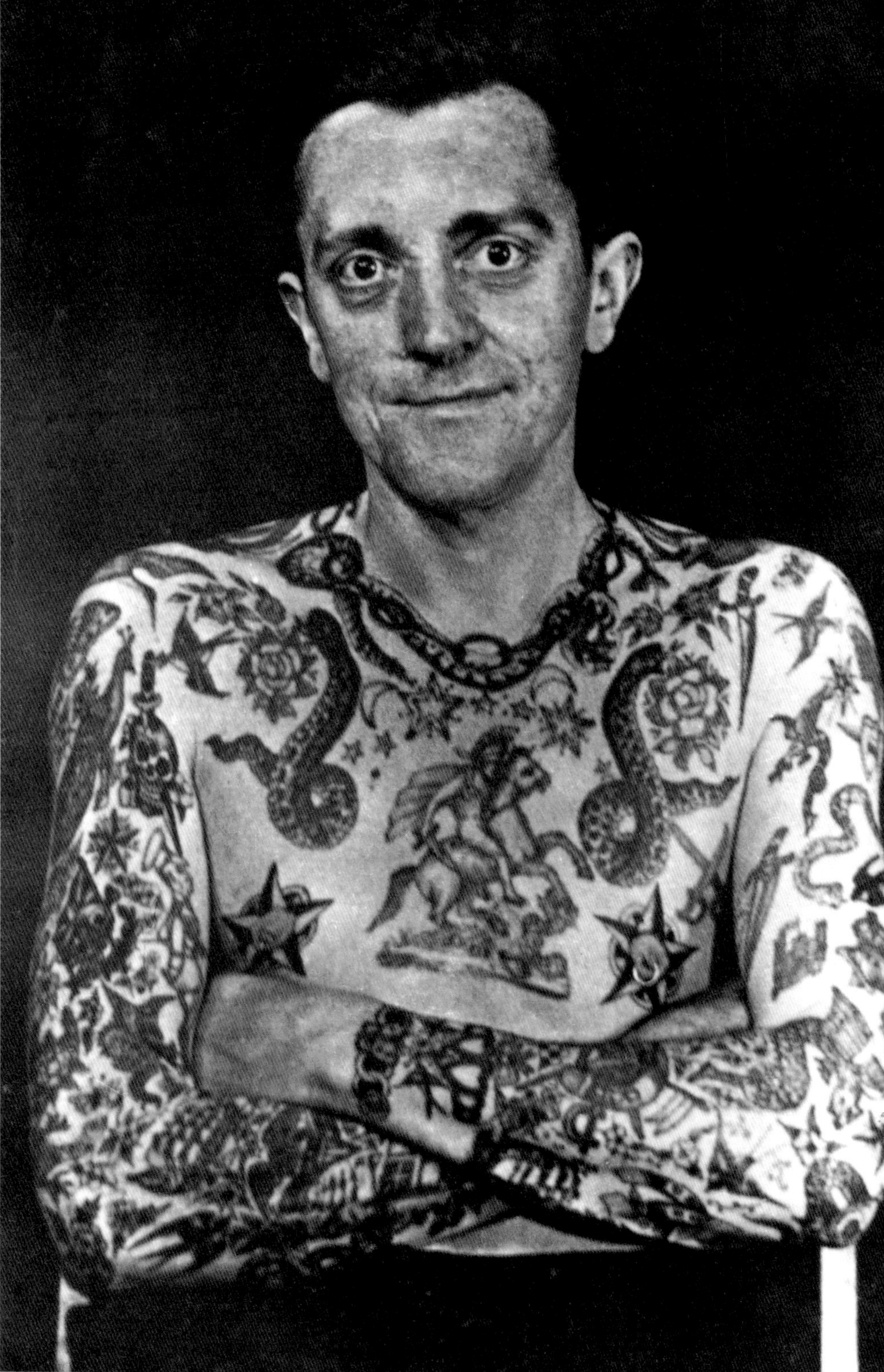

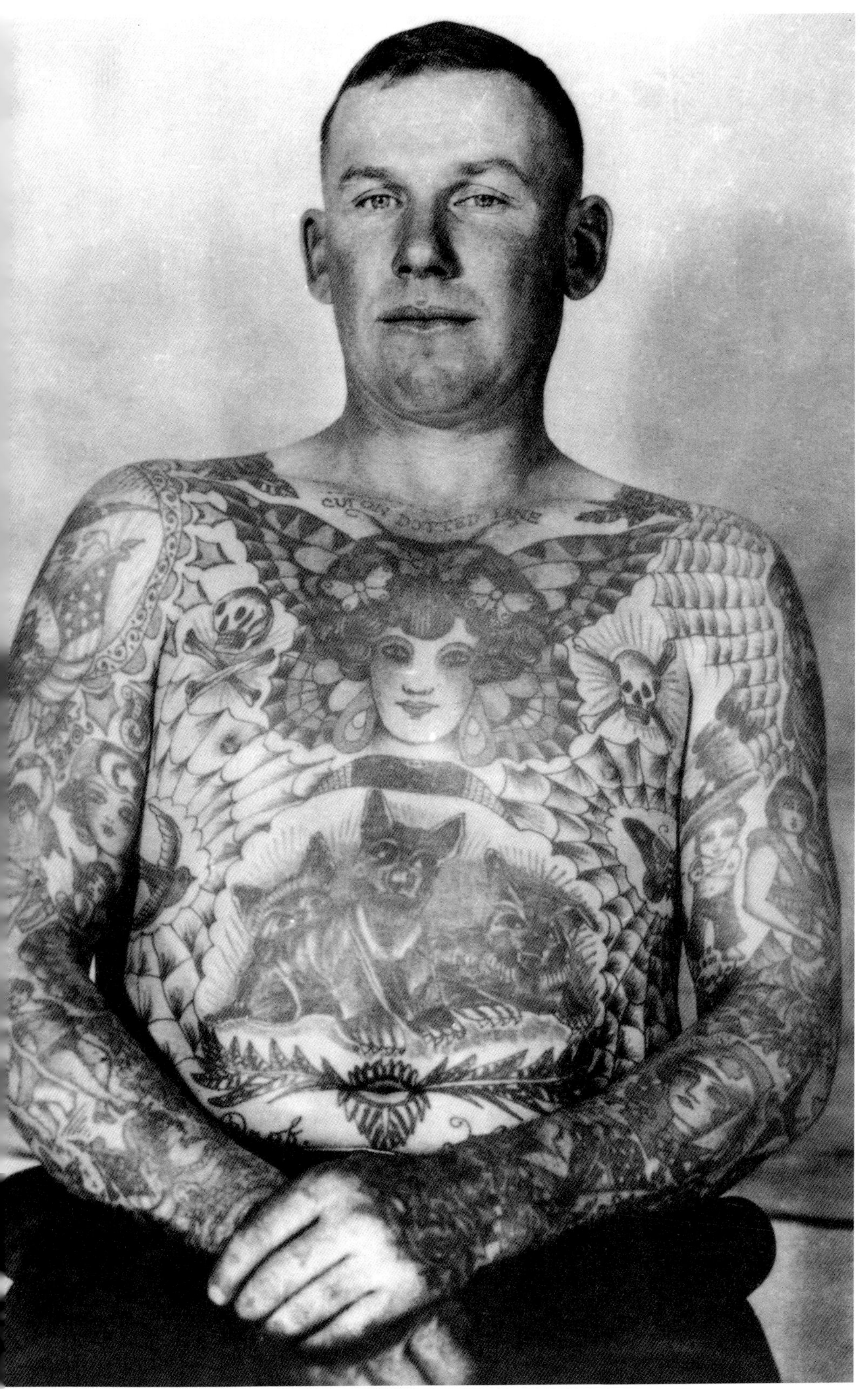

CUT ON DOTTED LINE

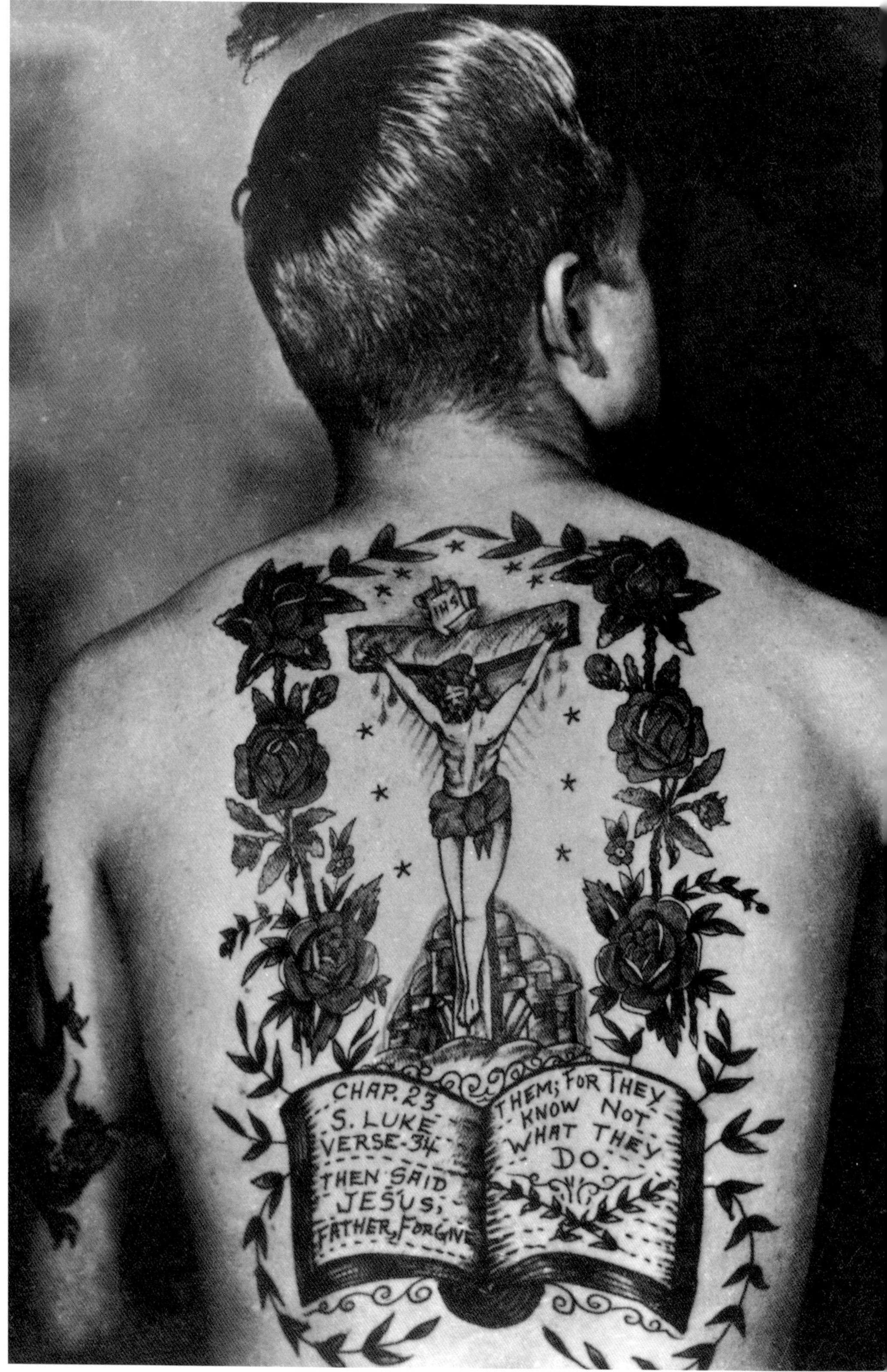
IHS
CHAP. 23
S. LUKE
VERSE - 34
THEN SAID
JESUS;
FATHER, FORGIVE
THEM; FOR THEY
KNOW NOT
WHAT THEY
DO.